The Yoga Back Book

By the same author:

Easy Pregnancy with Yoga

The Yoga Back Book

Stella Weller

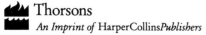
Thorsons
An Imprint of HarperCollins*Publishers*

Thorsons
An Imprint of HarperCollins*Publishers*
77-85 Fulham Palace Road,
Hammersmith, London W6 8JB

Published by Thorsons 1993
10 9 8 7 6 5

A catalogue record for this book
is available from the British Library

ISBN 0 7225 2785 3

Typeset by Harper Phototypesetters Limited,
Northampton, England
Printed in Great Britain

Contents

Acknowledgements

I thank all those who have contributed to this book through their encouragement and expertise. In particular, I am grateful to Jane Bowden for her splendid illustrations; Dr W. Harry Fahrni for reading the manuscript; John Hardaker of John Hardaker Editorial Services for his wise counsel and for reliably representing me; Judith Kendra, Veronica Simpson and Erica Smith of Thorsons and my husband, Walter Weller, for his unfailing support.

Introduction

Back problems have become epidemic. Almost every one of us will experience some form of backache or pain or related symptom at some stage of our life. Many of us will subject ourselves to unnecessary, ineffective treatments or give up activities we enjoy. Back problems, moreover, have become extremely costly: they result in absenteeism from work and they generate incalculable misery.

And yet according to experts, the care and management of our back is essentially *our* responsibility, and self-treatment of low back pain and similar problems brings better and more lasting results, in the long term, than any other form of therapy.

For more than four decades I have lived a full and highly productive life, despite a marked lateral curvature of the spine (scoliosis). I attribute this, in large part, to the observation and practice of principles of back care which I now share with you in this book. These are based on the ancient wisdom of yoga – a system of non-strenuous exercises done with full awareness, in synchronization with appropriate breathing, and special mental and respiratory exercises that promote relaxation and help in coping with stress.

Yoga, which was tremendously popular in the 1960s and 70s, is now making a strong comeback. I believe this is because of people's disenchantment with the unfulfilled promises of many high-impact, aerobic-type exercises and the potential of some of them for injury. Yoga is ideal for the millions of people who suffer from backache and related problems. Its gentle movements and the concentration and synchronized breathing it requires make it impossible to hurt yourself, provided the rules are adhered to. One eminent orthopaedic specialist has written, in fact, that as controlled stretching exercise yoga has no peer, and that the mental and physical discipline involved in its practice is superb (Abraham, 191). Other authors of books on back care have devoted entire chapters to exercises to which they refer as 'similar to yoga', an acknowledgement of the respect with which the yoga system is regarded.

This book is intended not only for those of you who are plagued with back problems, but also for those of the privileged minority who aren't and who wish to keep it that way. It can also be a useful reference for health care professionals such as doctors, nurses, physiotherapists and fitness instructors. It emphasizes personal responsibility in the management of back problems. It also stresses prevention, and provides the tools to help forestall difficulties and maintain the health of the spine and related structures. These tools include information on how the vertebral column is constructed, how to use it intelligently and how to care for it through a sensible balance of appropriate exercises, relaxation and sound nutrition.

Sixty illustrations complement clear instructions for performing the exercises correctly and safely. These include not only back exercises but also exercises for the legs and abdomen, which are crucial to the health of the back. An entire chapter has been devoted to the principles of good body mechanics, knowledge of which is vital to the prevention of back injury. Yet another chapter focuses on the special needs of those with problems such as chronic fatigue and difficulty with sex, while useful direction is given to pre- and post-natal women.

Hippocrates, known as the father of medicine, emphasized prevention and an awareness of the whole person when treating illness. An important part of this emphasis was the education and encourage-ment of patients to take responsibility in assisting the therapist with their own care. *The Yoga Back Book* does just that, and provides information and instruction for helping put those principles into safe, pleasurable practice to bring about the desired results.

Chapter 1

Back Basics

Before driving a car or using a piece of machinery, people usually acquaint themselves with the way it works. This allows them to operate it intelligently and therefore safely. The human spine, which is perhaps more sophisticated in its design than most machines, should be similarly considered.

A basic understanding of how the spine is constructed and how it functions is therefore a vital first step toward acquiring and maintaining a trouble-free back. This chapter represents that important first step. Spend a few minutes reading it from beginning to end. The time you invest in so doing will be rewarding: it will equip you to care for your back with insight and wisdom.

Functions and structure

The spine supports the head and about 90 per cent of the weight of the human body in an upright position. It is mechanically balanced to conform to the stress of gravity and to permit movement from place to place, as well as to assist in purposeful movements.

The spine prevents shock to the brain and spinal cord during activities such as running and jumping, through its curves and intervertebral discs, about which more information will be given later. It protects the spinal cord, which it houses. It provides attachment for many powerful muscles, and

it forms a strong posterior boundary for the body.

Known also as the spinal or vertebral column, the spine is composed of 33 bones

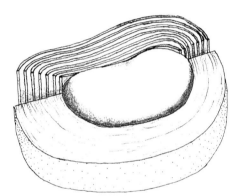

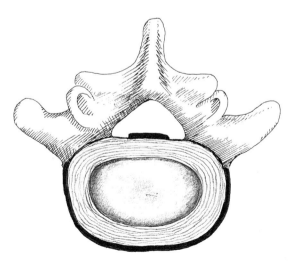

Fig. 1 *Intervertebral disc*

11

(vertebrae; singular, vertebra) with a pad of cartilage, or gristle (intervertebral disc) in between every two bones (Fig. 1). This disc buffers the vertebrae against shock during activities such as running, jumping or driving on bumpy roads.

The discs

The disc has a tough elastic shell composed of crisscrossing fibres. Inside it (the nucleus) is a soft substance with the consistency of jelly. The upper and lower surfaces of the disc have a cartilaginous layer known as an end plate. This acts somewhat like a sieve between the disc and the bone.

Discs have no blood supply; they depend on a process of diffusion through the end plates for their nutrition. When we are resting or sleeping, the discs suck in water and other nutrients. When we move about or exercise, compression squeezes fluids

out and expels wastes. A sensible balance of exercise and rest is therefore crucial in maintaining the health of the intervertebral discs.

All individuals can expect degenerative changes in the discs. Between the ages of 20 and 30, maximum development of the discs has occurred and the water content is maximal – about 80 per cent. This lessens with age. With a healthful lifestyle, however, it is possible to keep the discs from drying out, and to preserve a good balance between fibre and fluid, even into advanced age.

Spinal units

You may also think of the spine as being composed of a number of functional units. Each unit (Fig. 2) consists of two segments: an anterior (front) portion which may be considered a hydraulic, weight-bearing, shock-absorbing structure comprising two vertebrae with a disc in between them, and a posterior (back) portion which may be thought of as a guiding mechanism. This includes three projecting pieces of bone: two projecting sideways and one rearward. You may be able to feel these as 'buttons' down the middle of your back. These processes provide for the attachment of ligaments and muscles.

In addition, the rear portion of the vertebra has two upper and two lower surfaces called facets. The lower facets of one vertebra glide along those of the vertebra below. The facets thus guide and limit the motion of one vertebra relative to its neighbouring vertebra.

The articulated posterior processes of the vertebrae form a canal which houses and protects the spinal cord. This is a bundle of nerve fibres connecting the brain with all parts of the body, and which carries messages to and from the brain.

On each side of the spine, between every

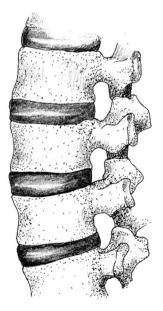

Fig. 2 Vertebrae with intervening discs

two vertebrae, are tiny openings for the passage of nerves branching from the spinal cord.

Ligaments and muscles

Strengthening the joints formed by the vertebrae and their intervening discs are ligaments ~ tough fibrous bands of tissue ~ running behind and in front of them along the entire length of the spine.

Reinforcement is also provided by the back muscles which help to control forward bending, and indirectly by the abdominal ('tummy') muscles which give a counter-balancing effect and help prevent extreme backward bending.

It is worth noting that although the abdominal muscles are not directly attached to the spine, their strength and tone are crucial to the overall health of the back.

Connective tissue

The spaces between the bones, tendons, ligaments and muscles of the back are filled with material known as connective tissue. Much of this filling is composed of a protein substance known as *collagen*. In fact, collagen accounts for about 30 per cent of total body protein. It is a sort of 'cement', which binds cells together. It is the key to the relationship between nutrition and spinal health. It acts as a transport medium, carrying nutrients from the bloodstream to the muscles and ligaments, and conveying wastes to the bowel and skin for elimination (Turner,102).

The chief functions of connective tissue in the back are: to bind tendons to bones and buffer muscles and ligaments to help maintain resilience and strength; and to act as a medium of transport, carrying oxygen and nutrients to spinal structures and removing wastes.

Spinal curves

With your mind's eye now, try to see the spinal column from the side (laterally). You will note four curves (Fig. 3): in the neck (cervical) region, one that is convex toward the front (lordosis); in the chest (thoracic) area, one that is convex toward the rear (kyphosis); at waist level (lumbar spine) another arch that is convex toward the front, and at hip level (sacral area) another arch that is convex toward the rear. These curves transect the plumb line of gravity in order to maintain a state of balance.

The pelvic ring

The spine is balanced on an undulating pelvic base known as the pelvic ring (sometimes the pelvic girdle). (Fig. 4). This is the human body's chief weight-transmitting structure, connecting the upper body to the legs. It consists of the *sacrum* at the back, and two *innominate* (hip) *bones* which are connected to the *femurs* (thigh bones). Together, these bones form five joints: two *sacroiliac* joints at the base of the spine; two hip joints where the hip bones connect with the legs, and the *symphysis pubis* where the two hip bones join in front.

A key feature of the pelvic ring is its strong ligamentous support, which is especially important in weight bearing.

During normal standing or sitting, the ligaments of the sacroiliac joints and the pelvic ring are somewhat loose. When weight bearing occurs, however, the pressure exerted down through the spinal column causes the sacroiliac ligaments to tighten. This tightening alters the position of the pelvic ring from a loose, or neutral structure to one that makes for greater stability.

A second key characteristic of the pelvic ring is that its degree of tilt determines the quality of the curves in the spinal column

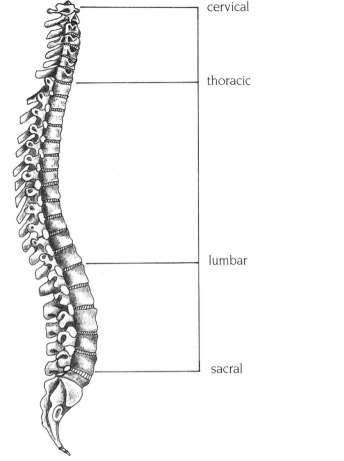

cervical

thoracic

lumbar

sacral

Fig. 3 *Spinal curves*

above. Any change in the angle of the sacral portion of the pelvis will influence the curves of the spine above, thus determining posture. If the pelvic ring is in a balanced position, the spinal curves will be proportionately balanced and the posture safe. If, however, the pelvic ring is abnormally tilted, poor posture will result and the spine will consequently be more vulnerable to injury and pain.

Good posture and smooth movement and rhythm require good coordination between nerves and muscles, good flexibility of tissues and adequate functioning of all joints involved.

Muscular supports

The chief back muscles are as follows. The *erector spinae* muscles form two columns, one on each side of the spine. They extend the spine and keep the trunk erect.

The *latissimus dorsi* is a broad, flat muscle lying over the lower part of the chest and loins (between ribs and hip bones). It draws the upper bone of the arm (humerus) down and back, and rotates the arm inward.

The *gluteal muscles*, which form the buttocks, raise the trunk from a stooping to an erect position. They are also involved in leg motions.

The *sling muscles* (hip flexors) connect the transverse processes of the spine on the inside (the projecting pieces of bone mentioned in the section on 'spinal units'), cross the pelvic ring and attach to the thigh bones just below the hips. They are very important in the maintenance of upright posture.

The *lateral muscles* are situated between the ribcage and the pelvic ring. They extend from the lowest ribs to the hip area and legs.

Secondary supports

Muscles forming secondary supports to the spine are: the *quadriceps* (thigh muscles), which run down the front of the thighs and insert into the kneecaps or patellae, and serve to extend the knees; and the *hamstrings*, which are located at the back of the thighs, passing from the pelvic ring and inserting into the bones of the lower legs (tibiae and fibulae). The hamstrings flex the knees and extend the thighs.

Both sets of muscles – quadriceps and hamstrings – contribute to the tilt or balance of the pelvic ring, and so are important to good posture.

The abdominal muscles, which will be dealt with in chapter six, basically extend from the breastbone (sternum) to the symphysis pubis, on each side of the midline. Although thin, these muscles give extremely important support to the spine. They operate at a distance and so provide leverage.

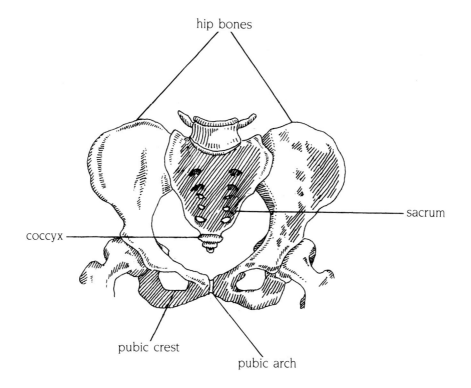

Fig. 4 *The pelvic ring*

Chapter 2

Body Moves

Postural patterns are influenced not only by lifestyle but also by genetic and early environmental factors. Without conscious, sustained effort, faulty postures can become permanent (Cailliet, 25).

There is no ideal posture, since people come in all shapes and sizes. The ideal posture for *you* is one in which your back is subjected to the least possible strain and in which the normal graceful curves of the spine are maintained (Tanner, 137).

The key to good posture is fitness. If you keep your muscles well conditioned, you stand a good chance of acquiring the posture that is correct for you, particularly if you complement this with a balanced mental and emotional state. This is the essence of the yoga approach.

Dr Bess Mensendieck, a sculptor turned physician, has remarked that correct posture, and freedom from pain due to faulty posture, can be acquired only when all muscles are used in accordance with their anatomical functions and with the laws of body mechanics. She has further noted that the primary exercise needed to achieve these states is the practice of correct postural habits during normal daily activities (Lagerwerff and Perlroth, 17). No daily half-hour exercise session alone will produce good posture if muscles and joints and related structures are not used properly the rest of the time.

A well-aligned vertebral column when we are upright or sit or lie down imposes the least strain on the spine. It is also an important prerequisite for the harmonious functioning of the nervous system, which is hinged on the backbone and the spinal cord, and for the free expansion of the chest to permit proper breathing. If we can maintain natural physical equilibrium when both sitting and standing, we minimize strain on the back muscles and facilitate harmonious distribution of the body weight along the 132 articulations of the vertebral column (Brena, 67-68).

In summary, your posture is determined by the way you hold each part of your body, from head to toes. Your posture affects your breathing, indeed your health in general ~ both physical and emotional ~ and the image you present to the world (Kounovsky, 11-12).

In order to relieve stress on the lumbar spine, a natural lumbar curvature, good balance and flexibility must be maintained at all times. The natural lumbar curvature is maintained through pelvic tilt (assisted by tightening abdominal and buttock muscles). This position distributes weight evenly down through the spine, allowing the strong leg muscles to bear the weight.

Now that you have a basic understanding of the structure and function of the spine, you will readily appreciate the principles of good body mechanics which follow, and the importance of maintaining the normal spinal curves.

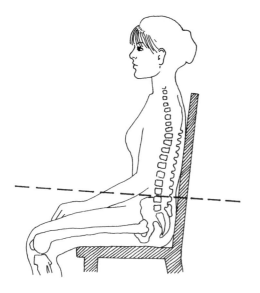

Fig. 5   *Good posture in sitting*

Sitting

Good posture when sitting puts the pelvis in a neutral position, that is, neither tilted backward nor tilted forward (remember that posture is controlled mainly from the pelvis).

The spine should be supported along its natural curve. The height of the seat should be such as to place the knees level with, or higher than, the hips (Fig. 5).

Figures 6 and 7 are examples of poor posture in sitting. In Fig. 6, the pelvis is tilted backward. This flattens the normal curve of the lower spine, stretching ligaments and eventually producing pain.

In Fig. 7, the pelvis is tilted forward, thus distorting good posture in much the same way as prolonged standing does. This, too, can lead to back strain and pain.

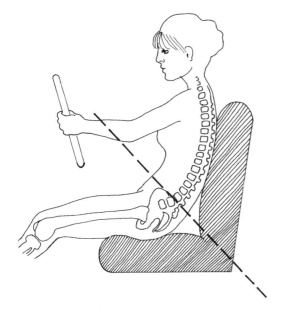

Fig. 6   *Poor posture in sitting*

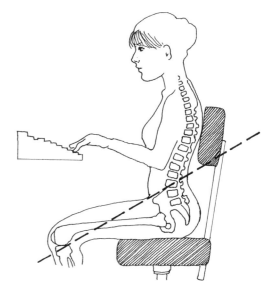

Fig. 7   *Poor posture in sitting*

The Easy Pose

One excellent way to sit is in the yoga *Easy Pose* (Fig. 8). It provides a stable base, encourages you to hold your spine naturally erect and promotes relaxation of the back muscles. It brings into play the sartorius, or tailor, muscles which lie across the thighs, from about the front of the hip bones to what we know as the shin bones. These are the muscles used in bending the legs and turning them inward.

Here's how to do the *Easy Pose*.

1. Sit with your legs stretched out in front.

2. Bend one leg and place the foot under the opposite thigh.

3. Bend the other leg and place the foot under the other bent leg.

4. Rest your palms quietly on the respective knees or place them upturned, one in the other, in your lap.

5. Maintain this position as long as you comfortably can, breathing regularly, and keeping your body relaxed.

Note

If your knees do not touch the surface on which you are sitting, do not be discouraged. They eventually will as your joints become more flexible and your ligaments more elastic.

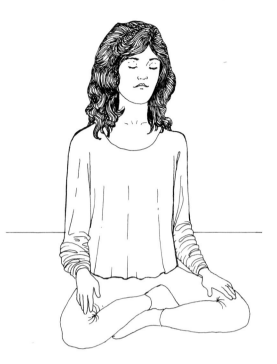
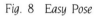

Fig. 8 Easy Pose

The Japanese Sitting Position

Here's another position that encourages good posture in sitting (Fig. 9).

1. Kneel down with your legs together and your body erect but not rigid. Let your feet point straight backward.

2. Slowly lower your body to sit on your heels. Rest your palms quietly on the respective knees. Sit tall and breathe regularly. Keep as relaxed as you can.

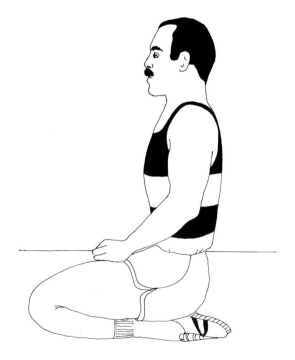

Fig. 9 Japanese Sitting Position

Note

If at first your heels cannot bear your weight, place a cushion between your bottom and heels, and hold the position only briefly. As your knees and ankles become more flexible and your body more conditioned, you will be able to sit in this posture for a longer time.

Squatting

One quarter of the human race habitually take weight off its feet by squatting (Cailliet, 23). A deep squat position for work and rest is used by millions of people in Africa, Asia and Latin America.

Squatting reduces any exaggerated curve of the lower spine, thus lessening tension in spinal muscles and ligaments. It reduces pressure on the spinal discs. As a result, the back is both strengthened and relaxed, and back discomforts are minimized. Squatting is, moreover, excellent for strengthening the ankles and feet.

The Squatting Pose

1. Stand with your legs comfortably apart. Distribute your body weight equally between your feet. Breathe regularly.

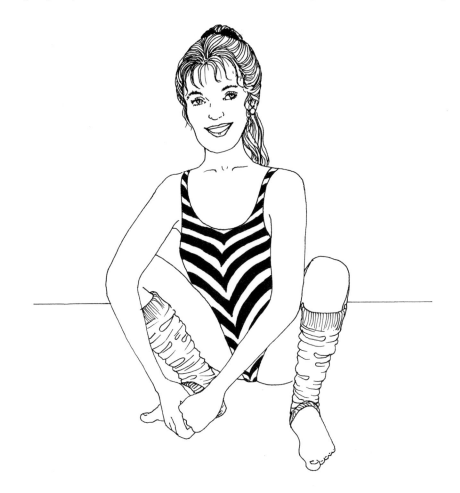

Fig. 10 Squatting Pose

2. Slowly bend your knees, lowering your bottom until you are sitting on your heels. Relax your arms for maximum comfort (Fig. 10). Hold this position as long as you can, breathing regularly.

3. Resume your starting position. Rest.

Note well

If you have varicose veins, you would do better to practise the dynamic version of the Squatting Pose which follows, rather than hold the squat for any length of time.

The Squatting Pose ~ Dynamic version

1. Stand with legs apart and arms at your sides. Inhale and slowly raise your arms to shoulder level as you simultaneously raise yourself on your toes. (If you have difficulty keeping your balance, use a stable prop for support.)

2. Exhale and slowly lower your arms as you lower your body into the squatting position (Fig. 10).

3. Without holding the position, come up again on tiptoe, repeating steps 1 and 2 several times in smooth succession, as many times as you wish. Relax afterwards.

This up-and-down version of the Squatting Pose gives a gentle, therapeutic massage to the legs and stimulates the blood circulation.

Sitting to prevent backache

● Sitting puts great pressure on spinal discs. Take periodic breaks from prolonged sitting to practise stretching and relaxation exercises. Two examples will be given later in this chapter.

● Be sure that the seat on which you habitually sit to do your work is well designed. It should be fully adjustable to suit your own measurements. It should support your back and legs comfortably. It should be at a height that permits you to do your work without having to stretch your arms forward from the shoulders. It should be adequately padded yet firm.

You might consider using a desk or other work surface that slopes towards you, so that you don't have to bend your head and neck down.

● **Do** arrange things on your desk so as to avoid having to twist back and forth.

● **Don't** cradle the telephone between your ear and shoulder. It promotes upper back tension.

● **Do** rest your arms on armrests when they're available.

● **Do** consider using a lumbar roll (back log), which is a support specially designed for the low back. Use it to good advantage when reading, writing, watching television or driving your car to counteract any tendency to slouch (McKenzie, 24). An ordinary cushion is not to be relied upon for long-term use; only in an emergency.

Back Break

To relieve back tension which builds up during prolonged sitting, a 'back break' is ideal. Get up from your seat and practise exercises to counteract the forward-bending attitude inherent in most sedentary activities.

Practise neck and shoulder exercises such as described in chapter four. Also practise a standing version of the Stick Posture (also chapter four), which is an excellent all-body stretch.

In addition, practise the two exercises to

follow. Modify them to suit your needs or circumstances.

Posture Clasp

1. Sit on your heels, in the Japanese Sitting Position (*see* Fig. 9). Breathe regularly.

2. Reach over your *right shoulder* with your *right hand.* Keep your elbow pointing upward rather than forward, and your arm close to your ear.

3. With your left hand, reach behind your back, from below, and interlock the fingers with those of the right hand. Maintain a naturally erect posture throughout the exercise, and keep breathing regularly (Fig. 11).

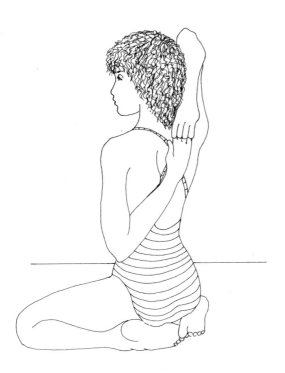

Fig. 11   Posture Clasp

4. Hold this position as long as you comfortably can. *Do not* hold your breath.

5. Resume your beginning position. Relax. Shrug your shoulders a few times, or rotate them, as you wish.

6. Repeat steps 2 to 5, changing the position of the arms and hands.

Variations

- You can practise the Posture Clasp in a standing position, or sitting on a stool or bench, or in a folded-leg position.

- If your hands don't touch each other, use a scarf or other suitable item as an extension: toss one end over your shoulder, and reach behind and below to grasp the other end. Pull upward with the upper hand and downward with the lower.

Chest Expander

1. Stand tall with your feet comfortably apart and your arms at your sides. Breathe regularly.

2. Inhale and raise your arms sideways to shoulder level; turn your palms downward.

3. Exhale and lower your arms. Swing them behind you and interlace the fingers of one hand with those of the other. Maintain a naturally erect posture and keep breathing regularly.

4. With fingers still interlaced, raise your arms upward to their comfortable limit; keep them straight (Fig. 12). Remember to maintain an erect standing position and to keep breathing regularly.

5. Hold this position as long as you can with absolute comfort. *Do not* hold your breath.

6. Slowly lower your arms, unlock your fingers and relax. You may shrug or rotate your shoulders a few times.

Standing

When we talk of poor posture, we generally mean slack posture. To correct this, there may be a tendency to cultivate posture that is excessively rigid, and this could result in tense muscles and restricted breathing.

In correct standing, the chin is in, the head up (crown uppermost), the back flattened and the pelvis straight (neutral position). The rib cage is full and round to permit adequate ventilation of the lungs and to prevent pressure on internal organs (Fig. 13).

In a strained position (Fig. 14), the pelvis tilts forward, thus increasing the spinal curves and strain on joints and ligaments. The chin is out and the ribs are down, causing pressure on internal organs. The lower back is arched (swayback). This is the most common type of poor posture in a standing position.

Even when standing correctly, there is tremendous pressure on lumbar discs - about 182 pounds per square inch on the third lumbar disc. Avoid standing, therefore, if you can sit, walk or squat. When you must stand, rest one foot on a convenient prop such as a bar rail, a box, a low stool or a shelf under a counter.

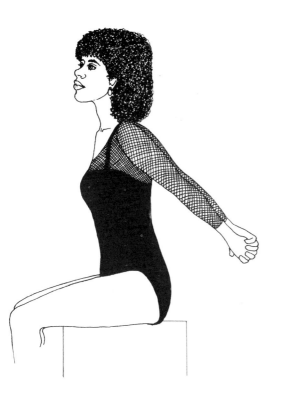

Fig. 12 Chest Expander

Variations

- Practise the Chest Expander in any comfortable sitting position.

- From step 4 above, continue thus: Slowly bend forward, keeping your back straight and bending at your hip joints rather than at your waist. Keep your arms pushed upward. Relax your neck.

  Hold the forward bend briefly, then slowly and carefully return to your starting position. Relax. (Did you remember to keep breathing regularly?)

Walking

Stand tall to reduce stress. Relax your shoulders. Flatten your shoulderblades. Tighten your abdominal and buttock muscles to help tuck your bottom in. Distribute your body weight equally between your feet. Breathe regularly. Swing your arms effortlessly. Move your legs from your hip joints. Practise Rhythmic Breathing (*see* chapter 8) for part of your walk.

When walking up stairs, try this: Plant the whole foot on the stair instead of walking on tiptoe. It will exercise your ankle and help conserve energy as you reach the top of the stairs.

23

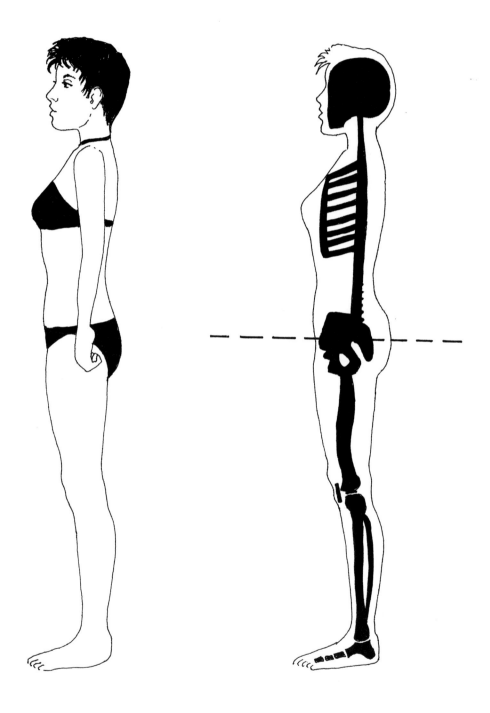

Fig. 13 *Good posture in standing*

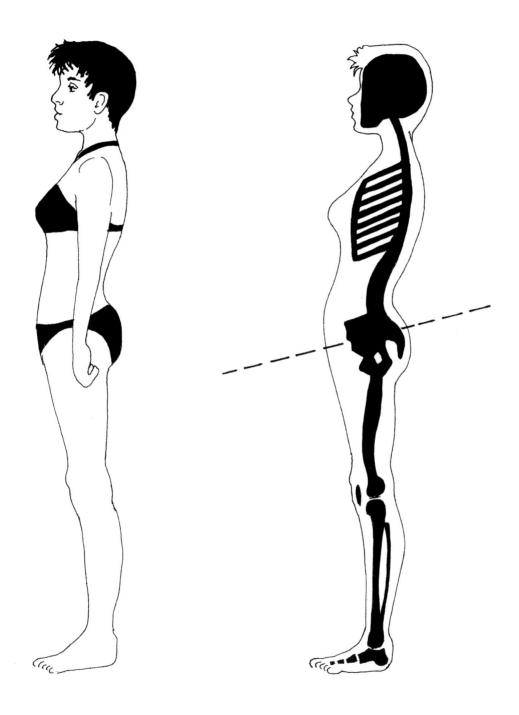

Fig. 14   *Poor posture in standing*

Lying

When you lie down, you relieve your spine of much of your body weight. This reduces compression on the discs. Experiment with lying positions to find those that are most restful for you.

Lie either on your back (supine) or on your side. Avoid lying on your abdomen (prone), as it places unnecessary strain on your lower spine. When you do have to lie prone, however, place a small pillow or cushion under your hips. It will prevent exaggeration of the spinal arch and reduce tension of the back muscles.

In the supine position, you can bend your knees and rest the soles of your feet flat on the surface on which you are lying. You may experiment with inserting a large cushion, pillow or bolster under the bent knees (Fig. 15). This is a very relaxing position for the back - one recommended by many orthopaedic specialists.

I sometimes lie in a similar position, but with my knees together and bent, soles flat on the mat or sofa or bed, and feet about the width of the hips apart. I find this easier to maintain for a longer time than if the knees were apart.

To counteract neck strain resulting from too much looking downward, try rolling a towel, like a sausage, and putting it under your neck as you lie on your back for half-an-hour or so. You may also arrange the rolled towel like a collar to prevent your head rolling to the side.

Consider using a feather or kapok pillow, which moulds itself to the contour of the head and neck while giving support and promoting relaxation. A foam pillow, by contrast, has recoil which tends to produce a certain amount of neck tension.

Your mattress should be firm yet able to conform to your body's contour without sagging.

When lying on your side, place a small pillow or cushion between your knees to prevent your hips from rotating and your spine from twisting. Both legs, or only the top one, may be bent for maximum comfort (Fig. 16).

Getting up (from lying)

Never get up in a rush. Avoid getting straight upward from a supine position. Instead, roll onto your side, bend your knees, bring them closer to your chest and use your hands to help push you onto your hip (Fig. 17).

Slowly pivot yourself until you are sitting evenly on your bottom, then slowly stand

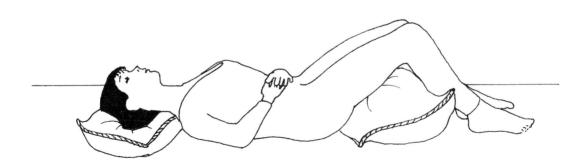

Fig. 15   *Good posture in lying (supine)*

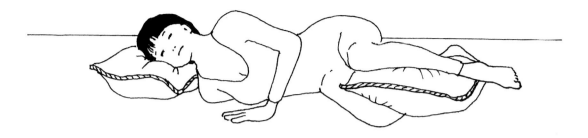

Fig. 16 *Good posture in lying (on the side)*

up. Breathe regularly all the while, to help you concentrate on what you are doing.

Carrying

To carry anything heavy ~ groceries, for example ~ divide them into two parts of roughly equal weight and carry one part on each side. Alternatively, look for someone to help you or use a trolley or cart if one is available.

Use luggage trolleys or wheels, or cases with wheels when you travel. Carry a small suitcase in each hand rather than struggle with a single large suitcase. Push trolleys rather than pull them to prevent back strain.

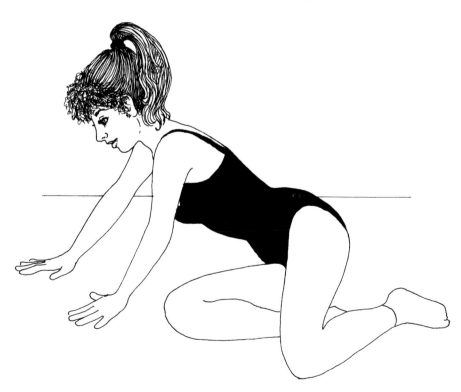

Fig. 17 *Getting up safely*

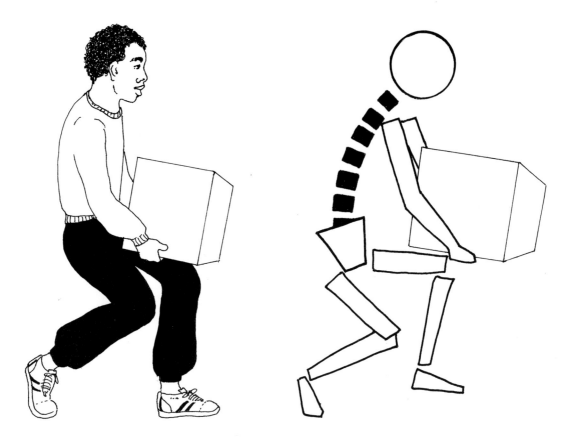

Fig. 18   Good posture in bending

Maintain good posture at all times and check that you are *not* holding your breath. Remember to keep breathing regularly.

Bending and lifting

Improper bending and reassuming a standing position is one of the most frequent causes of low back pain.

You can protect your spine when lifting by holding the object close to you with both hands to prevent the body from being pulled into the poor forward-leaning posture and also to prevent twisting. Good balance and flexibility are maintained by placing the feet in a broad-based stance and by bending the knees. This stance allows the body to move as a unit, and the weight to be shifted from one leg to the other (Caruth and Thompson, 6-7).

To avoid subjecting your back to unnecessary stress and to prevent injury, observe the following basic steps when bending and lifting.

1. Keep your back straight but not necessarily vertical. Bend your legs and lower yourself as if to squat.

2. For best balance, position your feet about

shoulder-width apart, with one in front of the other. The forward foot should be flat and the rear on tiptoe, as it were. Your knee should not touch the floor (Fig. 18).

3. Securely grasp the object to be lifted. Bring it close to you. Keep your arms close to your body.

4. Get up slowly and with awareness, letting the powerful leg muscles work for you. Observe good posture. Breathe regularly.

Avoiding pitfalls

Here are more tips to help prevent back injury when you bend and lift.

● Prepare the setting and the equipment. Render your work area safe by removing clutter, or by noting any unevenness or slipperiness of terrain, for example. Make sure there is adequate space in which to move.

● Wear suitable clothing which permits ease of movement, and which won't get caught or cause other impediment.

● Prepare your posture: place your feet apart in a walking stance. Bend your knees. Tighten your abdominal muscles. Maintain the neutral pelvic tilt (see Fig. 13). Use both hands. Hold the object close to you.

● Before lifting an object, be sure that you have a secure grip on it; use aids if necessary, such as slings, ropes or a mechanical lift.

● Concentrate on what you are doing (*see* chapter eight for concentration exercises). Breathe regularly.

Reaching

Avoid back strain through overreaching. To get something from a high shelf, stand on a stable stepladder or sturdy piece of furniture so you can reach the object with ease. If you feel insecure, hold on to something safe with one hand.

Concentrate when stepping up and stepping down. Breathing regularly will help you focus attention on what you are doing.

Vacuuming, mopping, shovelling, etc.

If your equipment is sufficiently lightweight, try using a lunging technique (Fig. 19) which will exercise the joints and muscles of your hips and legs. These, remember, are secondary back supports (*see* chapter one) which contribute to the health of the spine.

Remember to keep the back naturally straight and to breathe regularly.

If you're shovelling earth or snow, face the area you're going to dig and point the forward foot in that direction. Keep your arms close to your body. Point the rear foot towards the place where the shovelful is to be deposited and turn from the hip (rather than the waist) towards the rear foot. (Fig. 20).

Catching

Try to avoid catching falling objects. Your muscles need time to contract sufficiently to protect spinal joints, ligaments and discs. If they have to contract suddenly, without ample warning, they may not be able to coordinate adequately and the force involved in catching may be enough to cause damage. You may also slip and fall.

In summary

Whether you sit, stand or walk, lie down or get up, bend, reach, lift or carry, your key to

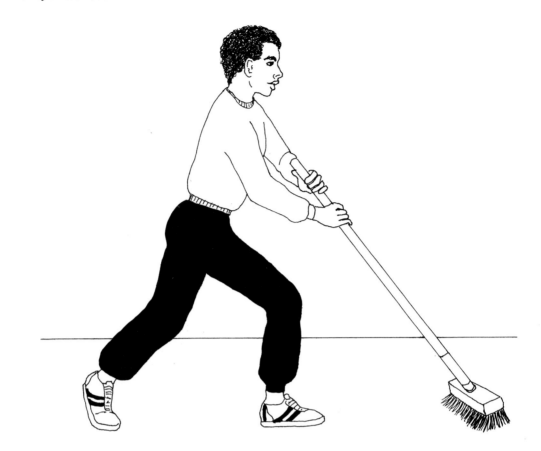

Fig. 19 Lunging

good posture is maintaining the normal curves of the spine. Any position, gesture, action or movement that alters these curves has the potential to place strain on spinal structures, weaken them, produce discomfort or pain and make the back more vulnerable to injury.

In order to maintain normal spinal curves, you need to keep your back, abdominal and leg muscles in good tone and you need to guard against overweight. You also need to balance regular exercise with rest and relaxation.

It is not only sedentary workers who need exercise. Even those whose occupations involve physical labour may be using certain muscles habitually to the neglect of others. Suitable exercises, done regularly, will help stretch out shortened muscles which contribute to poor posture. Exercise will help keep joints freely movable and less liable to be injured. Examples of such exercises are given throughout this book.

Please remember to *check with your doctor* before practising these or any other exercises. Ask if they are suitable for *you*, and compatible with treatment you may be receiving.

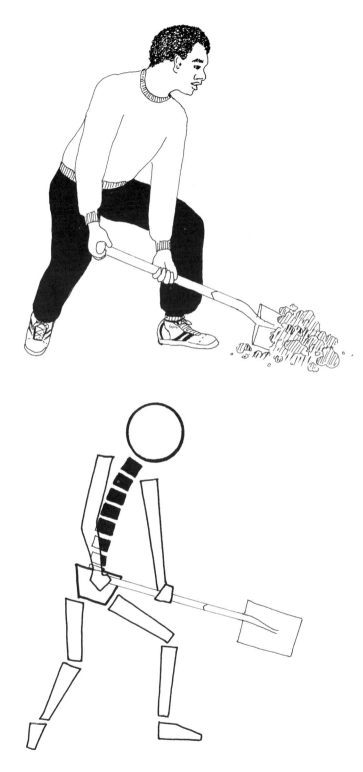

Fig. 20 Shovelling

Chapter 3

Diet for a Healthy Back

To stay alive and to function optimally, all living tissue needs oxygen and nutrients. The circulation through which these vital substances are delivered to the tissues must also be healthy. If the blood supply is reduced because of muscle spasm or poor posture, for example, then the nutrition to the affected parts of the body will be diminished and their function will be impaired.

It is essentially what we eat that provides the body with the raw material for building and maintaining a healthy spine, spinal discs, muscles, connective tissues and other components of the system. Nutrients from an adequate, wholesome diet are processed by the digestive system and transported to all cells and tissues through the blood circulation.

This chapter does not offer yet another fad diet. It simply highlights nutrients that are crucial to the structure and function of the spine and its attachments. It suggests sources from which to obtain these nutrients, and alerts you to substances that work against them. Although I have focused on only a few, it is well to remember that *all* nutrients work together and that no single one can be considered a panacea.

Vitamins

Vitamin A

This fat-soluble vitamin has a scavenging effect on *free radicals*, substances that are by-products of protein, carbohydrate and fat metabolism. They are considered 'mischievous molecules' which play a part in ageing and in cancer development. As such, vitamin A is a highly protective nutrient.

Cell oxygenation, whereby cells are supplied with oxygen, is enhanced by vitamin A combined with vitamin E.

Vitamin A increases permeability of blood capillaries which carry oxygen and other vital nutrients to the body's cells. (Capillary permeability exists when the capillary wall allows blood to pass readily into cells and tissue spaces and vice versa. The more permeable the capillary walls are, the better is the supply of oxygen delivered to cells.)

Vitamin A may play a part in protecting the linings of joints and so reduce the chances of inflammation.

The best vitamin A food sources are fresh vegetables, especially intensely green and yellow ones such as broccoli, carrots, dandelion leaves, kale, parsley, spinach and turnip leaves; fresh fruits such as apricots, cantaloupe melons, cherries, papaya and peaches; and milk, milk products and fish liver oils.

The B vitamins

Sometimes called 'the nerve vitamins', this complex contains more than twenty vitamins. They include thiamin (B_1), riboflavin (B_2), niacin (B_3), pyridoxine (B_6), folic acid (B_9) and cyanocobalamin (B_{12}).

The richest natural sources of the vitamin

B complex are brewer's yeast, legumes (dried peas, beans and lentils), whole grains and cereals, green leafy vegetables and wheatgerm.

Antistress factors

These are vitamin-like substances that protect against various stressors.

They are associated with the B vitamins and are found in green leafy vegetables, some nutritional yeasts, soy flour from which the oil has not been removed, and wheatgerm.

Vitamin C

This water-soluble vitamin is needed for healthy tissues, to promote healing and to reinforce resistance to disease. It must be supplied daily since it is not stored in the body.

Vitamin C is essential for the formation and maintenance of *collagen*, the strong cement-like material that holds cells together. As pointed out in chapter one, much of the protective connective tissue in the back is composed of collagen, which is formed largely of protein. Connective tissue plays an important role in the transport of nutrients to various structures (such as bones, tendons and muscles) and in the elimination of waste matter from them.

Vitamin C also contributes to the utilization of oxygen and to the maintenance of a healthy blood circulation. It is also an anti-stress vitamin.

The best vegetable sources of this vitamin are cabbage, dandelion leaves, green and red peppers, kohlrabi, mustard and cress and turnip tops.

The best fruit sources of vitamin C are apricots, blackberries, cantaloupe melons, cherries, elderberries, gooseberries, grapefruit, guavas, honeydew melons, kiwifruit, kumquats, lemons, limes, oranges, papayas and strawberries.

Rosehips are an excellent vitamin C source, also rich in *bioflavonoids*, which are substances that enhance the action of vitamin C.

Vitamin D

This fat-soluble vitamin facilitates the absorption and utilization of calcium, a mineral that is vital for healthy bones (more on this later).

Our most reliable source of vitamin D is vitamin D-enriched milk, not the action of sunshine on the skin, as was formerly believed.

Butter, eggs and fish liver oil contain small amounts of vitamin D. Plant foods contain none.

Vitamin E

This is another anti-stress vitamin, which also improves the circulation and averts certain types of oxygen damage to cells. Vitamin E, moreover, plays an important role in the transport, absorption and storage of vitamin A. It also protects against environmental influences, such as radiation, which destroys certain nutrients.

Good vitamin E sources include almonds and other nuts, broccoli, eggs, fresh fruits, green leafy vegetables, legumes, seeds, unrefined vegetable oils, wheatgerm and whole grains.

Minerals

Calcium

Calcium is an anti-stress mineral that is needed for sound bones and good muscle tone. It is also required for the proper functioning of nervous tissue and for normal blood clotting.

Bone is composed of very hard, dense tissue that is basically made up of an outer compact layer and an inner spongy matrix. This inner bone matrix consists of collagen fibres with deposits of calcium salts, magnesium and sodium – minerals that are constantly being stored or mobilized to meet the body's needs. A calcium deficiency could, understandably, result in weak bones that are vulnerable to injury and disease.

Calcium is known to relieve muscle cramps. In fact, the late Adelle Davis, author of several bestsellers on nutrition and health, referred to calcium as having the potential to be as soothing as a mother and as relaxing as a sedative. As such, it is useful for promoting sound sleep, which many backache sufferers find elusive.

Emotional stress and lack of exercise increase the need for calcium.

Milk is our best and most readily absorbed source of calcium, but if you are concerned about your fat intake, you can use skimmed milk, skimmed milk yogurt and buttermilk.

Another point in favour of milk as a calcium source is that it has a calcium to phosphorus ratio of five to four, which is nearly perfect for calcium absorption.

Some people, however, cannot tolerate milk, cheese and other dairy foods. They are lactose intolerant, which means that they either do not make the enzymes needed to digest milk sugar or they do not make enough of them.

For these individuals, there are certain products on the market (LactAid is one) which, when added to milk, break down the lactose, making the milk acceptable to the digestive system.

There are also non-dairy calcium sources which include canned salmon and sardines with the bones left in; almonds, beans, blackstrap molasses, broccoli, carob powder, citrus fruits, dried figs, some green leafy vegetables such as bok choy and spring greens (collards), sesame seeds and tofu (soy bean curd).

Calcium supplements, available at chemists and health food stores, may be the answer for those who are not taking in adequate amounts of this mineral through their diets. These supplements include calcium carbonate products and calcium lactate.

Vitamin D intake must be adequate for calcium absorption to take place. Vitamin C enhances its absorption.

Recipe: High-calcium shake

Here's a recipe for a beverage that's rich in vitamin D, calcium, silica, fluorine and other important bone-strengthening nutrients. It's easy to make and it's enough for one person.

Into an electric blender pour a cup of chilled, low-fat, vitamin D-enriched milk. Add one tablespoon of low-fat powdered milk, a teaspoon of unpasteurized honey, a few drops of pure vanilla extract and a few fresh strawberries (washed, and from which the caps and stems have been removed).

Blend the ingredients for a few seconds or until you have a smooth, frothy milk shake.

Boosting calcium intake

● Try figs for snacks. One fig contains 23 milligrams of calcium. (Figs, however, are high in calories.)

● Sprinkle stir-fried broccoli with toasted almonds or grated Parmesan cheese.

● Use yogurt as a base for dips, spreads and toppings.

● Try tofu in lasagna and stir-fried dishes.

● Use almonds or cheese cubes in salads.

● Use milk instead of 'whiteners' in tea and coffee.

Osteoporosis

Osteoporosis is a condition in which the bones become thin due to a lack of calcium in the bone matrix. (Bone matrix is the intercellular substance from which bone tissue develops.) The weakened bones may then break easily.

Poor nutrition over time or poor assimilation of nutrients are major factors contributing to osteoporosis. Usually thought of as a disease of old age, osteoporosis may, however, begin decades before – as early as twenty-five in some individuals.

With osteoporosis, prevention is better than treatment. Exercise, along with adequate calcium, silica, vitamin D and fluoride intake, will help to prevent it.

To remineralize damaged bones, you might consider supplementing your diet with organic vegetal silica dissolved in half a glass of lukewarm water and sipped slowly. The suggested dose is one or two teaspoons daily. Do, however, *check with your naturopathic physician or other therapist*. More information on silica is given later in this chapter.

Fluorine

This mineral works with calcium to strengthen bones (and teeth). The fluoride added to drinking water is sodium fluoride; it is not the same as calcium fluoride which is natural. (The former, taken excessively, can be toxic.)

Organic fluorine is found in steel-cut oats, sunflower seeds, milk and cheese, carrots, garlic, beetroot tops, green vegetables and almonds. It is also normally present in sea water and in naturally hard water.

Magnesium

Magnesium is another anti-stress mineral. It is necessary for the synthesis of protein and for the metabolism of vitamin C and the minerals calcium, phosphorus, sodium and potassium. It is essential for the proper functioning of muscles and nerves.

As a supplement, magnesium is measured in milligrams (mg) and is usually included in multivitamin-mineral preparations. Some supplements have magnesium and calcium in perfect proportion; that is, half as much magnesium as calcium.

The best food sources of magnesium include alfalfa sprouts, almonds, apples, dark green and other fresh vegetables grown on mineral-rich soils, figs, grapefruit, lemons, oranges, peas, potatoes, soy beans and yellow corn.

Silica

Silica is an essential nutrient that must be constantly supplied from food sources. It plays an important part in many body functions and has a direct relationship to mineral absorption.

Bones are made up mainly of calcium, magnesium and phosphorus, but they also contain silica. Silica is essential for both the hardness and the flexibility of bones, and it is silica that is responsible for the depositing of minerals, especially calcium, into the bones. Moreover, silica hastens the healing of fractures and reduces scarring at fracture sites. Silica also contributes to the building-up of connective tissue, and a deficiency leads to its weakening.

Along with regular exercise, silica supplementation is well worth considering for the relief of aching and ageing joints, and to alleviate certain intestinal upsets which may be connected with lower back pain. Two to four organic flavonoid chelated silica tablets or organic vegetal silica capsules daily, with meals, is considered reasonable supplementation to silica-rich foods. *Check with your naturopathic physician or other therapist* for the dose that is right for you. Spring horsetail (*Equisetum arvense*), better known as horsetail or scouring rush, is a perennial that grows wild in temperate zones. It is a rich, natural source of organic silicates, from which vegetal silica is derived. Pure aqueous extract of vegetal silica from spring horsetail is 100 per cent water soluble, and can therefore be completely absorbed by the body. (*Caution*: Ground horsetail is *not* suitable as it can be abrasive to the intestinal tract.)

Foods rich in silica include barley, brown rice, corn, oats, millet, rye, sunflower seeds and whole wheat; fresh fruits and vegetables such as apples, cherries, pears, strawberries; asparagus, red and green peppers, celery, green leafy vegetables, Jerusalem artichoke, kale, lettuce, onions, parsley, potatoes and red beets.

Other nutrients

Water

Water is the most important substance we consume. It is the principal constituent of body fluids and the medium by which nutrients are transported to all cells and wastes removed from the system. It is a shock absorber and a lubricant. The spinal discs are about 80 per cent water (*see* chapter one).

Water is the best drink for replacing fluid lost from tissues. This is because it quickly empties from the stomach, unless it is sweetened with glucose or other sugar.

Protein

Protein forms the basic structure of all cells, and a deficiency will result in loss of muscle mass and tone.

Protein is essential for the synthesis of collagen (*see* chapter one). Collagen represents about 30 per cent of total body protein.

An excess of protein, however, is undesirable. It increases the need for other nutrients, such as the B vitamins. A high-protein diet may result in increased calcium excretion through the urine, and therefore less calcium in the bones.

Legumes, nuts, seeds and grains such as corn, millet, oats and wheat are some of the best vegetable protein sources.

Amino acids

Amino acids are protein building-blocks. In recent years, researchers have demonstrated that the body also uses amino acids to help ease pain, relieve stress, help curb appetite and induce and prolong sleep – all important considerations for people with back problems.

Care must be taken when supplementing with amino acids. They must be perfectly balanced, since many of them work together in precise ratio. Please *consult a qualified nutritional counsellor* before taking amino acid supplements.

All good quality proteins will provide you with dietary amino acids (*see* section on proteins).

Carbohydrates: complex versus simple

Natural complex carbohydrates, as provided by whole grain breads and pasta, fresh fruits and fresh corn and other vegetables, are rich in nutrients. They are more slowly released from the stomach than the simple carbohydrates obtained from refined foods such as white flour, white rice and white sugar.

Complex carbohydrates furnish bulk, which appeases appetite and counteracts constipation which sometimes leads to lower backache. Complex carbohydrates, moreover, contribute to a trim body, discouraging overweight and obesity, both of which are linked to back problems.

Many people falsely believe that a high-carbohydrate diet is fattening. The fact is, however, that a pound of steak has 1200 calories, which is more than the calories contained in an entire loaf of whole grain bread.

Tips for increasing complex carbohydrate intake

● Discard the notion that complex carbohydrate foods are fattening.

● For breakfast, try porridge or a high-fibre, low-sugar breakfast cereal. Add a sliced banana or other fresh fruit. If you wish to include something sweet, use sultanas or raisins. As part of your breakfast, eat a couple of thick slices of whole grain toast, but go lightly on the butter or margarine.

● For snacks, eat whole grain bread rolls, crispbreads, muffins, fresh fruits, fresh vegetables or even whole grain breakfast cereal.

● For lunch, eat a nutritious sandwich made of whole grain bread; or have a baked potato, baked beans, pasta, brown rice or some other whole grain food.

● For supper, make rice, pasta and vegetables the main part of the meal.

● For dessert, fresh fruit is best.

● Take care not to add too much fat of any kind to your food. Complex carbohydrates have less than half the calories of fat. They are unlikely to increase body weight unless they are eaten with a great deal of fat.

Nutrient antagonists

Agents that act against the potential good of the vitamins, minerals and other nutrients provided by the food you eat are known as antagonists. The most infamous of these are contraceptive pills; excessive use of caffeine, salt, sugar and alcohol; over-exposure to the sun and other forms of radiation; high stress levels and lack of regular exercise.

Other vitamin and mineral antagonists are aspirin, which increases the need for vitamin C; rancid foods, which destroy vitamin E; some commercial laxatives (such as those containing mineral oil), which lead to deficiencies of vitamin C and the B vitamins; smoking, which reduces oxygen supplies to the tissues and destroys the B vitamins and vitamin C, and high-protein diets, which may result in increased calcium excretion through the urine, leaving less calcium in the bones.

In a nutshell: Diet for a healthy back

● Eat liberally those foods which contain calcium, silica, fluorine, vitamin C and vitamin D.

● Avoid high-protein diets.

● Reduce your intake of high-fat foods.

● Increase your complex carbohydrate intake.

● Cut down on your caffeine and alcohol intake.

● Drink plenty of water.

● Be wary of nutrient antagonists.

● Shop wisely: build your meals around fresh fruits, fresh vegetables and whole grain products. Store and cook your purchases to conserve nutrients.

● Eat slowly to aid digestion; don't overeat.

Chapter 4

Warming Up and Cooling Down

Experts agree that regular, appropriate exercise is essential for the prevention of back problems and for preserving the health of the spine. Before doing exercises, however, adequate warming up is essential.

Warm-ups prepare the heart muscle for exercise. They stretch the skeletal muscles and help reduce stiffness. They increase body temperature and they improve blood and lymph circulation. They help prevent muscular pulls and strain once the main exercises are in progress.

The warm-up exercises which follow have been selected because they are simple yet effective for limbering up the body. Several of them are also useful as tension relievers. They help prevent a buildup of tension which could lead to aches and pains. These warm-ups can readily be incorporated into daily schedules. For example, the neck, shoulder and ankle exercises can be done during breaks from prolonged sitting at a desk or machine, or at stops at suitable rest areas along the way during a long car journey. The *Rock-and-Roll* exercise can be done on coming home from work, before tackling evening chores. Be on the lookout for opportunities to weave these and similar exercises into the pattern of your daily activities.

Before starting the warm-ups, however, please read the following instructions which apply to the practice of all the exercises in this book.

General instructions

The exercises in this book are to be done with awareness and synchronized with regular breathing. Practised this way, they are safe and very effective. Please, however, *check with your doctor* and obtain his or her permission to do them, so that you are confident that they are suitable for *you*, and compatible with any treatment you may be having. Modify the exercises, if necessary, to suit you personally, and discontinue them at the first hint of discomfort.

When you have to restart regular practice after a period of interruption, do so in a gradual way, starting with the simplest version and working toward the most challenging. *Don't* try to make up for lost time by overexerting yourself.

Try to practise daily but if this is not possible, practise every other day so as not to lose the benefits gained from your previous exercise session.

When to practise

Try to do your exercises at approximately the same time every day (or every other day) to establish a good habit.

Practising in the morning reduces stiffness resulting from hours of lying and gives energy for the day. Practising in the evening produces a healthy fatigue and promotes good quality sleep. If, however, you find evening exercise too stimulating, try to fit your exercises in where they prove most convenient and beneficial. Several of the exercises such as the neck, shoulder and ankle warm-ups, as well as many of the breathing exercises (*see* chapter eight) can be done at odd moments throughout your work day, to prevent tension from accumulating. For example, you can tighten your abdominal muscles on an *exhalation* when standing or sitting. You can rotate your ankles when watching television with your feet elevated. You can check your posture whenever you pass a mirror. You can do breathing exercises when driving or waiting in a queue (line-up) or at boring parties.

Whatever the time you choose for your exercise session, make sure that two or three hours have elapsed since you last ate, depending on the content and size of the meal. After practising, avoid eating for at least half an hour.

Before starting

Empty your bladder, and bowel if possible. If you are especially stiff, a warm (*not* hot) bath may prove useful. It's a good idea to brush your teeth and clean your tongue to enhance a feeling of well-being, and clear your nasal passages to permit easy breathing.

Where to practise

Choose a quiet, well-ventilated room with soft lighting in which to do your exercises. Arrange not to be interrupted as you practise, since concentration is essential when performing yoga exercises (asanas).

Whenever possible, try to practise outdoors, such as on a lawn or on a patio on which a mat is spread.

Remove from your person any object that may injure you, such as glasses, hair ornaments, jewellery, etc. Wear comfortable, lightweight clothing that permits ease of movement and respiration, and which allows your skin to breathe.

How to practise

One characteristic of many popular exercise programmes of the past was the ever-increasing number of times an exercise was repeated and the decrease in the resting interval between them. Relaxation, which is a significant component of muscle activity, was thus neglected (Noble, 81).

Multiple repetitions of an exercise tend to produce stiffness and fatigue. Instead of tiresome repetitions, therefore, you can come back to a specific exercise later, or try a more advanced variation of it, or experiment with different exercise combinations so that you exercise all muscle groups, or give extra attention to those that need more strengthening.

Periods of rest and breathing appropriately while exercising are as important as the exercise itself. Doing exercises slowly and with full awareness ensures control of your position and movement at all times and helps prevent injury. These principles are inherent in the yoga approach to exercise, an approach that represents centuries of wisdom.

When ready to do the exercises in chapters five, six and seven, pay attention to the following points, which are characteristic of all yoga exercises (also known as asanas, poses or postures).

● Always begin by warming up. Specimen warm-ups will follow.

● Exercise on a firm, even, well-padded surface. This will be referred to, from now on, as the 'mat'.

● Give full attention to what you are doing.

● Visualize the completed exercise. This is your goal, but not one that you must attain today. The attempt, as well as perseverance in practice, is what ultimately matters.

● Breathe regularly throughout each exercise. Do *not* hold your breath. Synchronize your breathing with the movement being performed. This permits delivery of oxygen to the working muscles and helps eliminate substances that cause fatigue.

● Except when doing warm-ups, in which several repetitions in smooth succession are usual practice, do the exercise once or twice only (you can repeat it later), making your movements slow and conscious.

● During the holding period (indicated as 'hold' in the exercise instructions), *do not* simultaneously hold your breath; keep the breath flowing.

● Always rest briefly after each exercise.

● At the end of your exercise session, be sure to cool down. Please refer to the section on cooling down later in this chapter.

Warm-up Exercises

The neck

The following exercises, done slowly and with awareness, in synchronization with regular breathing, are wonderful for keeping the cervical (neck) part of the spine flexible and healthy.

Figure-eight

Sit comfortably. Close your eyes or keep them open. Keep your shoulders, arms and hands relaxed. Breathe regularly throughout the exercise. Imagine a large figure-eight lying on its side in front of you. Starting at the middle, trace its outline with your nose or mouth, a few times in one direction. Pause briefly. Trace the outline of the figure-eight a few times in the other direction. Rest.

Ear-to-shoulder

Sit comfortably. Close your eyes or leave them open. Keep your shoulders, arms and

hands relaxed. Breathe regularly throughout the exercise. Tilt your head sideways, as if to touch your shoulder with your ear (Fig. 21).

Bring your head upright. Tilt your head toward the opposite shoulder. Bring your head upright. Repeat the exercise a few times in smooth succession.

Head rolls

Sit comfortably. Close your eyes or keep them open. Keep your shoulders, arms and hands relaxed. Breathe regularly throughout the exercise. Bend your head forward. Slowly, smoothly and carefully roll it to one side then backward until you feel a delightful stretch of the neck. Roll it to the other side then back to the front. Raise your head up. This is one rotation.

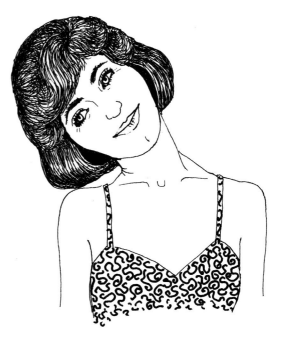

Fig. 21 Ear-to-shoulder exercise

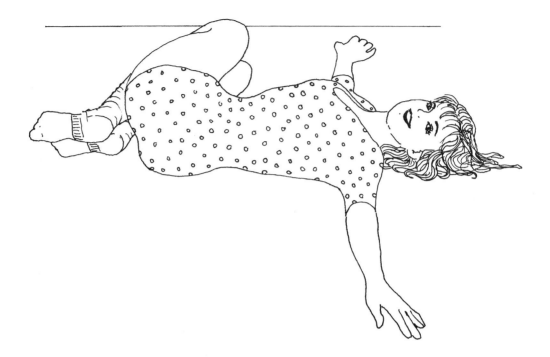

Fig. 22 Lying Twist

Repeat the rotation several times in slow, smooth succession, alert for any hint of discomfort. At the first suggestion of strain, stop the exercise. Rest after you have completed a few head rolls first in one direction, then a few in the opposite direction.

The shoulders

The following shoulder exercises enhance the effects of the preceding neck exercises, as well as conditioning the upper back.

Shrugging

Sit comfortably erect. Keep your head still and your eyes open or closed. Breathe regularly throughout the exercise.

Pull your shoulders upwards (shrug) as if to touch your ears with them. Hold the shrug briefly (*do not* hold your breath), then relax your shoulders. Repeat the exercise a few times.

Rotating

Sit comfortably erect. Keep your head still and your eyes open or closed. Breathe regularly throughout the exercise.

Pull your shoulders downward and backward, squeezing your shoulderblades together. Bring them forward and upward, then backward and downward to complete one rotation.

Repeat the rotation several times in smooth succession, then repeat the rotations a few times in reverse.

The Lying Twist

This is an exercise in torsion (twisting), which is beneficial to the abdominal muscles and to the lumbar part of the spine.

1. Lie on your back, with your arms sideways at shoulder level. Breathe regularly.

2. Bend your legs, one at a time, so that the soles of the feet are flat on the mat.

3. Bring the bent knees toward the chest.

4. Keeping the shoulders and arms in firm contact with the mat, *slowly, gently and smoothly* tilt the bent knees to one side as you exhale. You may keep your head still or you may turn it to the side opposite the tilted knees (Fig. 22).

5. Inhale and bring the knees back to the upright position, as in step 3.

6. Exhale and tilt the knees to the other side, keeping the head still or turning it opposite to the tilted knees, as preferred. Be sure to keep your shoulders pressed to the mat.

7. Repeat the side-to-side tilting of the knees, several times in slow, smooth succession.

8. Stretch out and rest.

Having worked from the neck downward, you are now ready to warm up the hip joints and legs. An excellent exercise for this is the *Butterfly*, and you will find it in chapter 7, Fig. 53.

The ankles

Rotating
Sit where you can move your feet freely. Observe good posture. Breathe regularly.

Rotate your ankles in slow, smooth circles. Repeat the rotations in the opposite direction.

Rock-and-roll

This is an excellent all-over warm-up that not only conditions the back and abdominal muscles, but also helps to loosen tight hamstrings. You may recall that the hamstring muscles, located at the back of the legs, contribute to the tilt of the pelvis and so are important contributors to good posture (*see* chapter one).

As an added benefit, when you practise the *Rock-and-roll*, you press on 64 traditional acupuncture points (Livingston, 39).

This exercise should be done on a firm, even, well-padded surface.

1. Sit on your mat. Bend your legs and place the soles of your feet flat on the mat, close to your bottom.

2. Pass your arms *under* your bent knees and hug your thighs. Tuck your head down and chin in; make your back as rounded as you comfortably can. Breathe regularly.

3. On an inhalation, kick backward to help you rotate onto your back (Fig. 23).

4. On an exhalation, kick forward to come up again into a sitting position. Do *not* land heavily onto your feet as this will jar your spine. Simply touch the mat lightly with your toes.

5. Repeat steps 3 and 4 several times in smooth succession, synchronizing your breathing with the rock-and-roll movements.

6. Sit or lie down and rest.

Fig. 23 Rock-and-roll (**Below**)

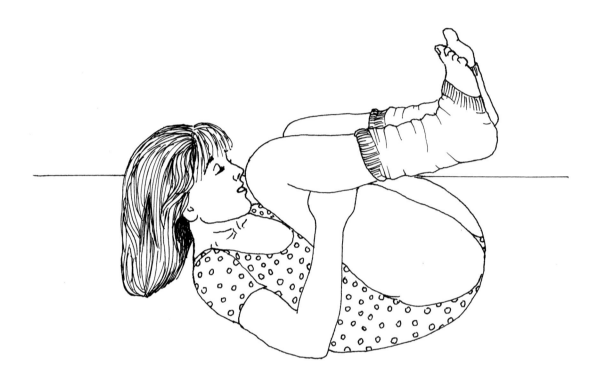

Sun Salutations

This sequence of yoga postures is particularly beneficial for the maintenance of all-round spinal health (Turner, 86). The twelve movements of the sequence exercise the spine forward and backward, and provide excellent leg stretches as well. They may be used not only as warm-ups but also as cool-down exercises.

1. Stand tall, with the palms of your hands together, as if in prayer (Fig. 24). Breathe regularly.

2. Inhale and carefully bend backwards to stretch the front of your body. Tighten your buttock muscles to help protect your back (Fig. 25).

3. Exhale and bend forward, at the hip joints rather than at the waist, and place your hands on the mat beside your feet (Fig. 26). If necessary, bend your knees; as you become more flexible you will be able to execute this step with knees straight.

4. Inhale and look up. Taking the weight of your body on both hands, step back with your left foot (toes point forward) (Fig. 27).

Fig. 24 (**Below**)

Fig. 25 (**Below**)

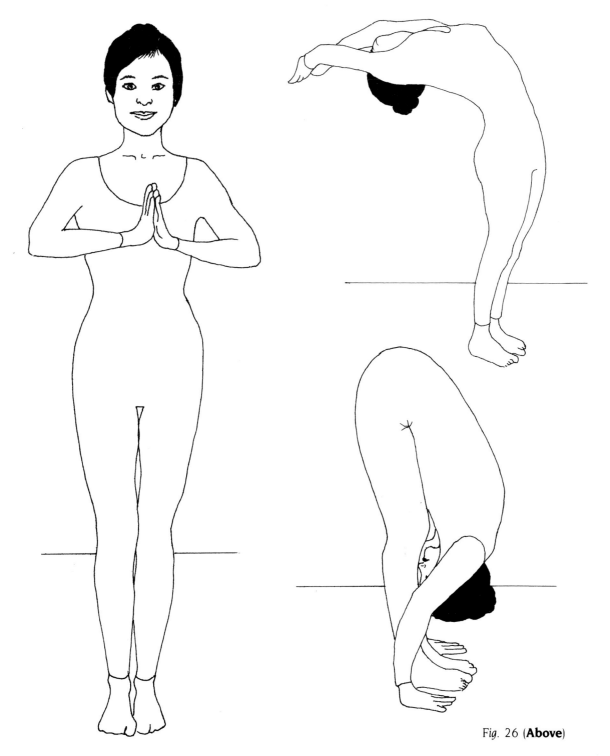

Fig. 26 (**Above**)

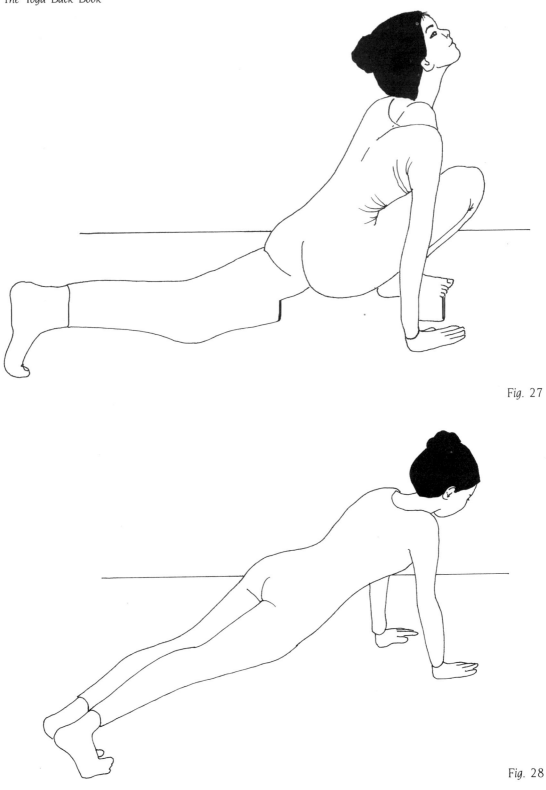

Fig. 27

Fig. 28

5. Briefly suspending your breath (neither inhaling nor exhaling), also step backward with your right foot. The weight of your body is now borne by your hands and feet, and your body is level from the back of your head to your heels (Fig. 28).

6. *Exhale* and lower your knees to the mat. Also lower your chin (or forehead – whichever is more comfortable) and chest to the mat (Fig. 29).

7. *Inhaling,* relax your feet so that your toes point backward. Lower your body to the mat and *slowly and carefully* arch your back. Keep your head up and back, and your hands pressed to the mat (Fig. 30). This is the *Cobra* position, which is again

described in chapter five in more detail, as a separate exercise.

8. *Exhale* and point your toes forward; push against the mat with your hands to help raise your hips. Arms are straight (or almost straight) and the head hangs down. Aim your heels toward the mat but *don't strain* (Fig. 31). This is the *Dog Stretch* position, which is again described in chapter seven as a separate exercise.

9. *Inhaling,* look up, rock forward onto your toes and step between your hands with your *left* foot (the same foot which you moved backward in step 4 of these instructions (Fig. 32).

10. *Exhaling,* step between your hands with your right foot and bend forward (as

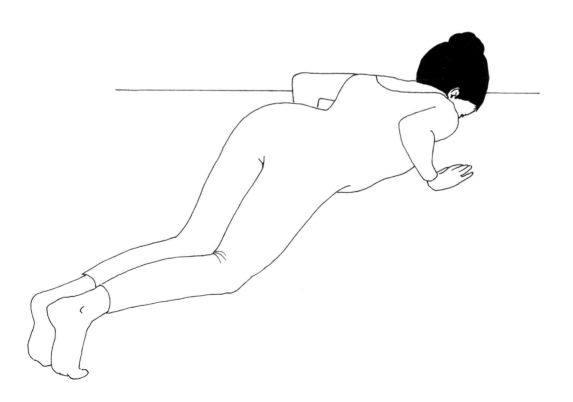

Fig. 29

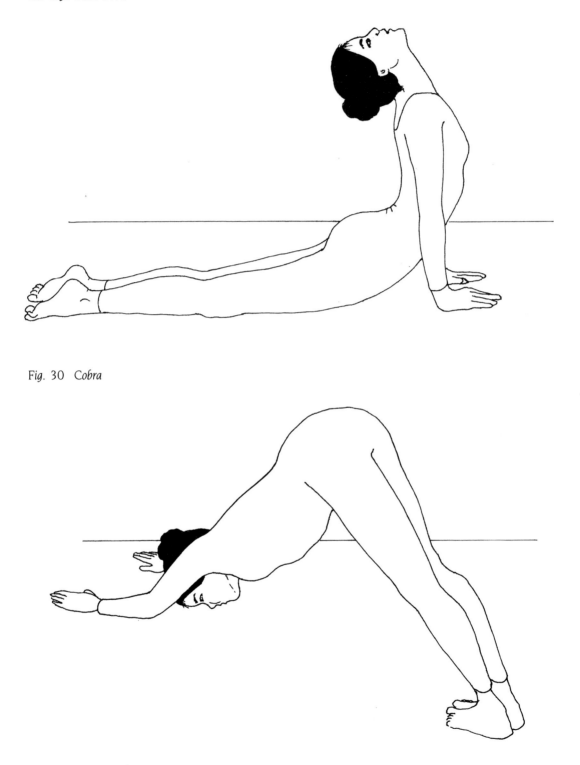

Fig. 30 Cobra

Fig. 31 Dog Stretch

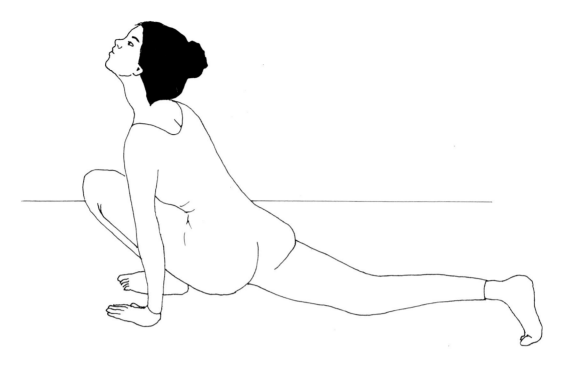

Fig. 32

described in step 3 of these instructions) (Fig. 26).

11. *Inhaling,* come up *carefully* into a standing position, and move smoothly into the backward bend described in step 2 of these instructions (Fig. 25).

12. *Exhaling,* resume your beginning position, as described in step 1 of these instructions (Fig. 24). Breathe regularly.

Repeat the sequence (steps 2 to 12) as many times as desired, alternating left foot with right in steps 4 and 9.

When you have completed these *Sun Salutations,* lie down and rest.

Cooling down

Cooling down after exercise affords a chance for static muscle stretching, which enhances flexibility. It provides an activity for the cardiovascular system (heart and blood vessels) to gradually return to normal functioning following exercise. It helps prevent problems such as a drop in blood pressure, dizziness and fainting, which can occur if exercise is stopped abruptly.

Most of the exercises given in the section on warm-ups can also be done as cool-down exercises. You may also wish to try the following.

The Stick Posture

This is essentially an all-over body stretch done in a supine, or lying on the back, position.

1. Lie on your mat, with your legs stretched out in front and your arms at your sides. Close your eyes and breathe regularly.

2. Inhale slowly, smoothly and deeply as

49

you bring your arms overhead and, if possible, place the palms together. At the same time, stretch your legs to their fullest extent, pulling your toes toward you and pushing your heels away from you.

The entire stretch should be one slow, smooth, conscious motion done in synchronization with your inhalation.

3. Hold the all-body stretch for seconds only, but *do not hold your breath*.

4. Exhale and release the all-over stretch, bringing your arms back to your sides, as in step 1.

5. You may repeat the exercise once, resting afterwards.

Toe-to-top relaxation (Savasana)

This exercise is a favourite of yoga students. It often marks the end of a yoga exercise session, and it is now frequently practised to promote deep relaxation.

The basic position is described in step 1, but you may modify this to suit *your* particular condition, preference or circumstances.

1. Lie on your back with your legs straight in front. Separate your feet to discourage a buildup of tension in the legs. Move your arms a little away from your sides to prevent an accumulation of tension in the shoulders. Keep the arms straight but relaxed, with the palms of the hands upturned. Close your eyes. Unclench your teeth to relax your jaws, but keep your mouth closed without compressing the lips. Breathe regularly (Fig. 33).

2. Focus your attention on your feet. Pull your toes toward you, pushing your heels away. Hold the ankle position briefly. Do *not* hold your breath. Keep breathing regularly throughout the exercise. Now relax your feet and ankles.

3. Stiffen your legs, locking your knee joints. Hold briefly. Relax your knees.

4. Tighten your buttock muscles. Hold the tightness for a few seconds. Release the tightness.

5. On an *exhalation*, press the small of your back (waist level) toward or against the mat. Hold the pressure as long as your exhalation lasts, then release the

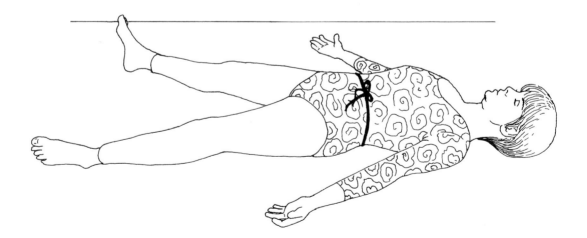

Fig. 33   Toe-to-top relaxation (Savasana)

pressure as you inhale. Keep breathing regularly.

6. Inhale and squeeze your shoulder-blades together. Hold the squeeze as long as the inhalation lasts. Release the squeeze as you exhale. Keep breathing regularly.

7. On an exhalation, tighten your abdominal muscles. Hold the tightness as long as the exhalation lasts. Inhale and relax. Keep breathing regularly.

8. Take a slow, smooth, deep inhalation, *without strain*, imagining that you are filling the top, middle and bottom of your lungs. Be aware of your chest expanding. Exhale slowly, smoothly and steadily, imagining that you are emptying your lungs by degrees. Be aware of your chest relaxing. Resume regular breathing.

9. Tighten your hands into fists; straighten your arms; raise them off the mat. Hold the stiffness briefly, then let the arms and hands fall to the mat, free of stiffness. Relax them.

10. Keep your arms relaxed, but shrug your shoulders as if to touch your ears with

them. Hold the shrug briefly, then relax your shoulders.

11. Gently roll your head from side to side a few times. Reposition your head. Keep breathing regularly.

12. Exhaling, open your eyes and mouth widely; stick your tongue out; tense all your facial muscles. Inhale, close your mouth and eyes and relax your facial muscles. Imagine your facial features becoming softer and more serene. Breathe regularly.

13. Lie relaxed for as many minutes as you can spare. Give your body weight up to the surface that supports it. Each time you exhale, let your body sink more deeply into that surface, increasingly relaxed.

14. Before getting up, rotate your ankles, roll your head gently from side to side, slowly and leisurely stretch your limbs, do the *Lying Twist* (Fig. 22), or whatever other gentle movements you feel like doing. *Never* get up suddenly. Get up carefully (*see* Fig. 17). Prepare to resume your usual activities, feeling wonderfully refreshed.

Chapter 5

Essential Back Exercises

In chapter one, you read about the anatomy of the spine and about other structures connected with it. All these components work together, in health, to keep you upright yet give you the flexibility to move about efficiently. They enable you to bend forward, backward and sideways, and to twist, or rotate, your body. They also allow you to turn your head in several directions.

The exercises that follow have been carefully selected to help strengthen the back and structures relating to it; to promote spinal flexibility; to keep joints freely movable and to relax back muscles. A rigid back is more vulnerable to pain, stress and injury than a flexible one. Faithful practice of these exercises is therefore encouraged.

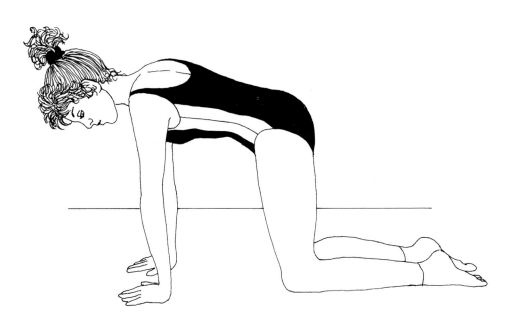

Fig. 34 Cat Stretch: 'All Fours' Position

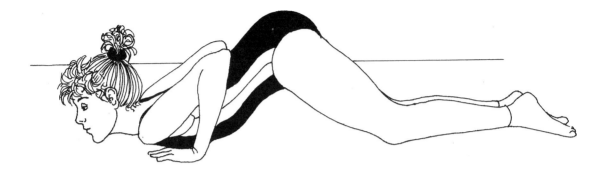

Fig. 35 Cat Stretch: 'Knee-chest' Position

Before starting

Before you begin to practise the back exercises in this chapter, please read the general instructions in chapter four and follow them.

Back Exercises

The Cat Stretch Series

1. Get on your hands and knees in an 'all fours' position (Fig. 34).

2. Inhaling, bend your elbows and lower your chest to the mat, taking care not to let your back sag. Keep your head back so that your neck receives a gentle, therapeutic stretch as your chin touches the mat. Let your arms and hands take most of the weight so as not to subject your back to unnecessary pressure. This is the 'knee-chest' position (Fig. 35).

3. On an exhalation, return to the all fours position described in step 1 (Fig. 34). Breathe regularly.

4. On an exhalation, lower your head, make your back rounded and bring one knee toward your forehead. This is the 'knee-to-forehead' position (Fig. 36).

5. Inhaling, push the bent leg backward, stretching it out fully and lifting it as high as absolutely comfortable; raise your head. This is the 'all-body stretch' (Fig. 37), which can be done without accentuating the inward curve of the back unnecessarily. Breathe regularly.

6. Exhale and lower your knee to the mat. Breathe regularly.

7. Repeat the all-body stretch described in step 5, with the other leg. Repeat step 6.

8. Lie down on your back and rest, or relax in the *Pose of a Child*, described later in this chapter (Fig. 45).

Note well

If you have recently given birth, *please check with your doctor* before practising step 2 (Fig. 35) of the Cat Stretch series. Done earlier than six weeks post-natally, you risk

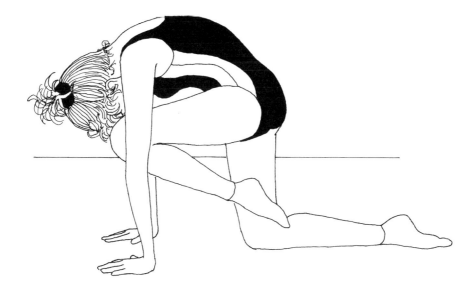

Fig. 36 Cat Stretch: 'Knee-to-forehead' Position

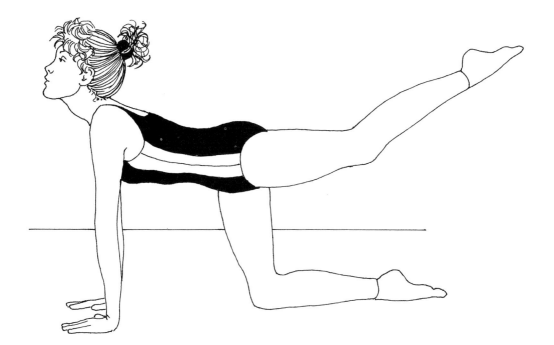

Fig. 37 Cat Stretch: 'All-body Stretch'

introducing air bubbles (air emboli) into your circulatory system.

The Pelvic Tilt Lying

1. Lie on your back with your legs outstretched in front.

2. Slide your hands under your waist. You will note a hollow – the lumbar arch of your spine (Fig. 38).

3. Now relax your arms and hands at your sides. Bend your legs and rest the soles of your feet flat on the mat, at a comfortable distance from your bottom. Breathe regularly. On an *exhalation*, press the small of your back (waist level) toward or against the mat to eliminate the hollow you felt there as you prepared for this exercise (Fig. 39). You will feel your pelvis tilt gently upward as you do this.

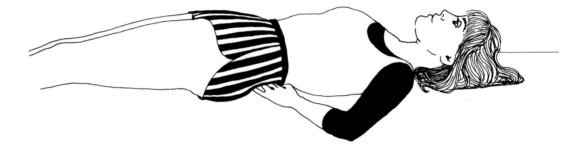

Fig. 38 *Preparing for the Pelvic Tilt Lying*

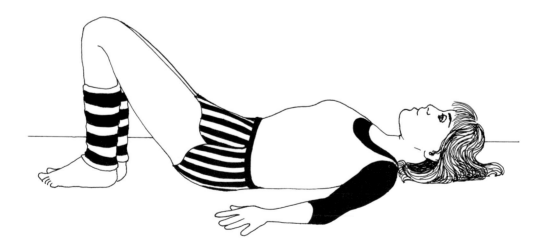

Fig. 39 *Pelvic Tilt Lying*

4. Hold the downward pressure of the waist as long as your exhalation lasts.

5. Inhale and relax.

6. You may repeat steps 3 and 4 once more now, and again later if you wish.

7. Stretch out and rest.

Variation: Pelvic Tilt on all fours

1. Get on all fours (Fig. 34). *Exhale* and tuck your bottom down. Lower your head. Make your back as rounded as possible.

2. Hold the position briefly, but *do not* hold your breath.

3. Inhale and resume your starting position, as in step 1. Breathe regularly.

4. You may repeat the exercise once now, and again later.

Variation: The Pelvic Tilt Sitting

1. Sit naturally erect on a chair with a straight back. Rest the soles of your feet on the floor.

2. On an *exhalation*, press the back of your waist firmly toward or against the back of the chair.

3. Hold the pressure as long as the exhalation lasts.

4. Inhale and relax. Breathe regularly.

5. You may repeat the exercise once now, and again later.

Variation: The Pelvic Tilt Standing

1. Stand naturally erect, with your back against a wall or other suitable prop.

2. *Exhale* and press the back of your waist toward or against the prop.

3. Hold the pressure as long as the exhalation lasts.

4. Inhale and relax.

5. You may repeat the exercise once now, and again later.

Notes
Opportunities for practising an appropriate version of the Pelvic Tilt are countless. Examples are: during television commercial breaks; while waiting for the kettle to boil; during breaks on a long car or bus journey; during tea or coffee breaks at your place of work (in the lounge, washroom or behind closed doors elsewhere in the building); against the wall of a lift (elevator) – no one will know what you're doing.

The Bridge

1. Lie on your back with your legs bent and the soles of your feet flat on the mat, comfortably close to your bottom. Relax your arms close to your sides, with your palms turned downward. Breathe regularly.

2. Inhaling, raise first your hips, then slowly and smoothly the middle of your back until your torso is off the mat (Fig. 40). Do *not* arch the small of your back (waist level) unnecessarily. Your feet, arms and hands, upper back and head remain in firm contact with the mat.

3. Hold the raised-torso position as long as comfortable, breathing regularly.

4. Slowly and smoothly lower your torso, *in reverse* motion, as if curling your spine, one bone at a time, onto the mat. Synchronize your breathing with this movement.

Knee Press

1. Lie on your back with your legs stretched out in front and your arms and hands relaxed beside you. Breathe regularly.

2. *Exhaling*, bend one leg and bring the bent

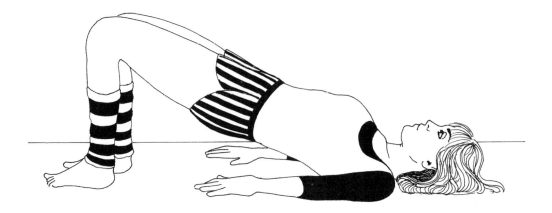

Fig. 40   The Bridge

knee toward you. Clasp your hands around the bent knee (Fig. 41). This is the basic knee press.

3. Hold the position as long as you wish, breathing regularly.

4. Return to the starting position, as in step 1.

5. Repeat steps 2 to 4 with the other leg.

6. Repeat the entire sequence (steps 2 to 5)

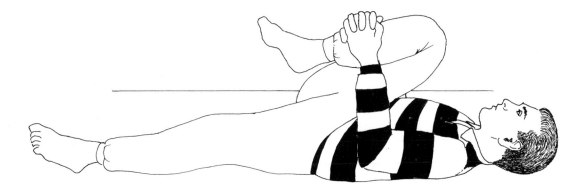

Fig. 41   Knee Press (Basic)

58

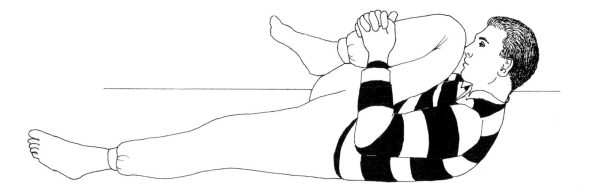

Fig. 42 *Knee Press (Variation I)*

once more now, and again later if you wish.

Knee Press (Variation I)

1. Lie on your back with your legs stretched out in front and your arms and hands relaxed beside you. Breathe regularly.

2. E*xhaling*, bend one leg and bring the knee toward you. Clasp your hands around the bent knee. *Carefully* raise your head and bring the forehead toward the bent knee (Fig. 42).

3. Hold the position as long as you wish, breathing regularly.

4. *Carefully* lower your head to the mat. Lower your leg to the mat, resuming your starting position, as in step 1.

5. Repeat steps 2 to 4 with the other leg.

6. Repeat the entire sequence (steps 2 to 5) once more now, and again later if you wish.

Knee Press (Variation II)

1. Lie on your back with your legs stretched out in front and your arms and hands relaxed beside you. Breathe regularly.

2. E*xhaling*, bend one leg and bring the knee toward you. Continue breathing regularly.

3. Again on an *exhalation*, bend your other leg and bring it toward you. Continue breathing regularly. Hold the bent legs securely.

4. *Carefully* raise your head and bring your forehead toward the bent knees as you *exhale*. Keep your shoulders as relaxed as possible (Fig. 43).

5. Hold the position as long as you comfortably can, breathing regularly.

6. *Carefully* lower your head to the mat.

7. Release the hold on each leg in turn and carefully lower it to the mat.

8. Rest, breathing regularly.

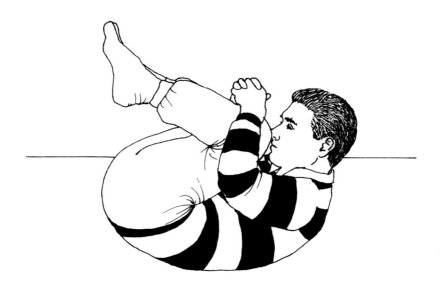

Fig. 43 Knee Press (Variation II)

The Star Posture

1. Sit comfortably erect, with your legs stretched out in front. Breathe regularly.

2. Bend one leg and place the sole of the foot flat on the mat, opposite the knee of the outstretched leg. (This establishes the distance to maintain between the feet and the rest of the body once you are performing the exercise).

3. Bend your outstretched leg. Place the two soles together.

4. Clasp your hands securely around your feet.

5. *Exhaling*, bend forward slowly, smoothly and with control, bringing your face toward your feet. Once you have reached your comfortable limit, relax your head downward (Fig. 44).

6. Hold the position as long as you are comfortable in it, breathing regularly.

7. Slowly resume your beginning position, synchronizing your movement with your breathing.

8. Lie down and rest.

The Cobra

This posture was described as part of the *Sun Salutations* (*see* chapter four, Fig. 30), but will be repeated here in more detail, as a separate exercise.

1. Lie on your abdomen, with your head turned to the side. Relax your arms and hands beside you. Breathe regularly.

2. Turn your head to the front, resting your forehead on the mat. Place the palms of your hands on the mat, directly beneath your shoulders. Keep your arms close to your sides.

3. On an *inhalation*, bend your neck backward, *slowly and carefully*: touch the mat with your nose then your chin in one smooth movement. Breathe regularly and continue arching the rest of your spine: the upper back then the lower back, again in one slow, smooth, graceful movement. Keep your hips in contact with the mat throughout the exercise. The completed *Cobra* is depicted in Fig. 30 in chapter 4.

4. When you can arch your back no further, hold the position, but *do not* hold your breath. Keep breathing regularly.

5. Come out of the position *in reverse, very slowly, smoothly and with control*: lower the abdomen to the mat; lower the chest,

chin, nose and forehead, in synchronization with regular breathing.

6. Relax your arms and hands beside you. Turn your head to the side. Rest.

Following the *Cobra*, get onto 'all fours' and thence into the *Pose of a Child* (Fig. 45), which follows.

Pose of a Child

1. Sit in the *Japanese Sitting Position* (*see* chapter 2, Fig. 9). Breathe regularly.

2. Slowly and carefully bend forward, resting your forehead on the mat, or turning your face to the side. Relax your arms and hands beside you (Fig. 45).

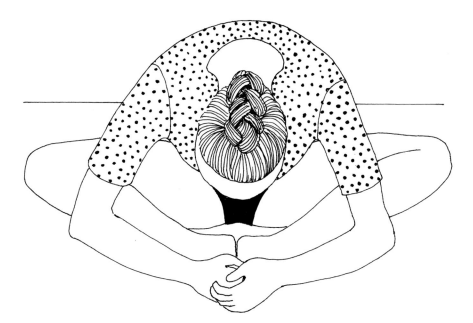

Fig. 44 Star Posture

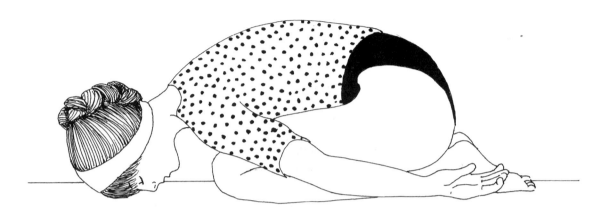

Fig. 45 Pose of a Child

3. Stay in this position as long as you feel comfortable in it. Continue breathing regularly.

4. Slowly resume your starting position, as in step 1.

Notes

● This is a good position in which to rest after backward bending poses such as the Cobra, chapter four, Fig. 30) and the Bridge, chapter five, Fig. 40).

● If you find that you can't get your head down to the mat, place a plump cushion or pillow in front of your knees, on which to rest your forehead or face.

The Half-Moon

1. Stand naturally erect, with your feet close together, and your body weight equally distributed between them. Breathe regularly.

2. Inhaling, bring your arms upward, pressing the palms together overhead if you can. Keep your arms aligned with your ears.

3. *Exhaling*, slowly and carefully bend to one side to form a gentle, graceful sideways arch of the body (Fig. 46).

4. Hold the position as long as you comfortably can, breathing regularly.

5. Inhale and return to the upright position. Exhale and lower your arms to your sides. Breathe regularly.

6. Repeat steps 2 to 5, bending to the other side.

7. Relax.

You may repeat steps 2 to 7 once more now, if you wish, and again later.

The Spinal Twist

1. Sit naturally erect on your mat, with your legs stretched out in front of you. Breathe regularly.

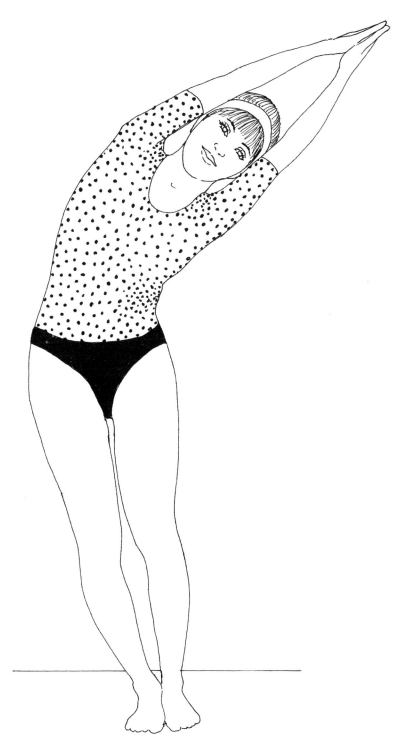

Fig. 46 Half-Moon

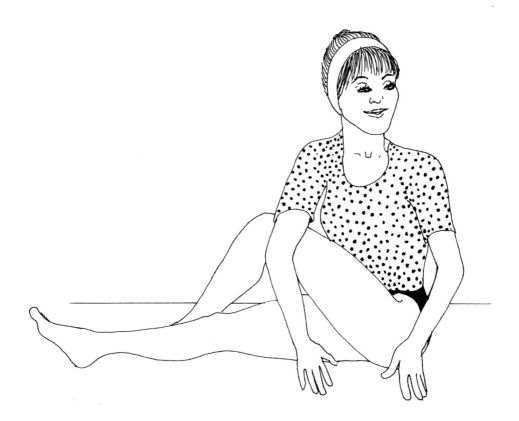

Fig. 47 Spinal Twist

2. Bend your *left* leg at the knee, and place the *left* foot beside the *outer* aspect of the right knee. Keep breathing regularly.

3. On an *exhalation, slowly and smoothly* twist your upper body to the *left*, and place both hands on the mat at your *left* side. Turn your head and look over your *left* shoulder (Fig. 47).

4. Hold the position as long as you comfortably can, but *do not* hold your breath. Keep breathing regularly.

5. *Slowly and smoothly* untwist and resume your beginning position, as in step 1.

6. Repeat steps 2 to 5 in the opposite direction (substitute the word 'right' for 'left' and vice versa in the instructions).

7. Relax.

Variations

When you become more flexible, you may wish to try this advanced version of the *Spinal Twist*.

1. Begin as in step 1 of the basic instructions just given.

2. Fold one leg inward, bringing the foot toward the upper thigh of the opposite, outstretched, leg.

3. Step over the folded leg with the other foot (when the left knee is uppermost, twist to the left; look over the left shoulder. When the right knee is uppermost, twist to the right; look over the right shoulder).

4. Repeat the twist in the opposite direction.

Rest afterwards. Remember to synchronize breathing with movement.

Pregnant women will welcome a gentler, more convenient spinal twist. You will find this described and illustrated in my book *Easy Pregnancy with Yoga* (*see* Bibliography).

To complete these essential back exercises, please also practise the *Half-Locust*, which is described and illustrated in chapter seven (Fig. 55).

Chapter 6

Abdominal Backing

Not everyone knows that the abdominal muscles provide backing, or reinforcement, to the muscles supporting the pelvis and spine. Many individuals will be surprised to learn that muscles located at the front of the body can actually be related to discomfort and pain felt in the back. In fact, lax abdominal muscles are a common cause of backache.

The abdominal corset

As mentioned in chapter one, in order to drive a motor vehicle or operate a piece of machinery intelligently you need some familiarity with its workings; in the same way, you can't appreciate the role of the abdominal muscles and the principles underlying abdominal exercises without at least a basic knowledge of the structure and function of these muscles.

Here, then, is a pain-free lesson in the positions, attachments and functions of the principal abdominal muscles, sometimes incorrectly referred to, even by health professionals, as the 'stomach muscles'.

The *rectus abdominis* (recti muscle) is a long, flat muscle that runs down the front of the abdomen, from the breastbone (sternum) to the pubic bones, on each side of an imaginary line drawn down the middle. It flexes the spine (as when bowing or bending forward), and it supports the viscera (organs inside the abdomen).

The *obliquus externus abdominis* is a muscle with fibres running obliquely from the lower ribs to the iliac crest, which some people can feel as the front of the 'hip bone'. It flexes the trunk laterally (sideways), rotates it (as when twisting) and it also supports the viscera.

The *obliquus internus abdominis muscle* is situated in the same place as the obliquus externus, but its fibres run in the opposite direction. These two sets of muscles are collaborators, working in harmony as one, to produce the same actions.

The *transversalis abdominis* lies beneath the two preceding muscles, and its fibres run transversely as its name suggests. It assists the oblique abdominal muscles, just mentioned.

Finally, there are the *quadratus lumborum* muscles, lying on each side of the vertebral column (spine), and running from the last ribs to the iliac crest in front. They help the other abdominal muscles perform their functions effectively.

The foregoing muscles are arranged like a four-way corset, spanning the front of the trunk from the breastbone and ribs to the pubic bones, and around the side of the ridge of the pelvis, which some people feel at each hip.

Although each muscle or set of muscles makes a contribution to the function of this abdominal corset, different sets work in combination during certain activities and exercises. For instance, the top half of the corset comes into play more noticeably than the bottom part during movements involving the upper trunk. When the legs are moved, however, it is the lower abdominals that are emphasized; they help stabilize the pelvis at this time.

Functions of the abdominal muscles

Here, for easy reference, is a summary of the functions of the muscles forming the four-way abdominal corset.

- To give support to the viscera (abdominal and pelvic organs).

- In collaboration with the buttock muscles (which pull downward as the abdominals pull upward), to control the tilt of the pelvis to maintain its correct alignment in relation to the spine.

- To flex the trunk sideways (half of the muscles are used).

- To raise the trunk upward from a supine (lying on the back) or semi-supine position; even raising the head will cause the abdominal muscles to tighten.

- To rotate the trunk, as in bringing one shoulder toward the hip on the opposite side.

- To help brace the body when it is being strained, as occurs during lifting or attempting to ward off blows. This is a reflex protective action.

- To help stabilize leg raising.

- To assist in conscious acts of breathing; in coughing, sneezing, shouting and singing, and in elimination of body wastes; also during childbirth.

It is worthy of note that sitting and standing postures provide little stimulus for abdominal muscles; nor does walking normally on level terrain. This is partly why the abdominals are usually the weakest group of muscles in people from industrialized societies. It is also partly the cause of the prevalence of backache: weak abdominals is one of the most common causes of backache. The abdominal muscles are afforded maximum exertion when they are required to perform against resistance, such as leverage and body weight. Other actions that effectively exercise the abdominals include trunk- and leg-raising from a horizontal position, running and lifting objects.

Essential principles for exercising abdominals

Before attempting practice of any abdominal exercise, it is a good idea to have some understanding of the principles underlying their action. Once you comprehend these principles, you will perform the exercises to follow more intelligently and therefore more safely; you will incur less risk of straining joints and muscles than if you practised in random fashion. You will also better appreciate chapter two, which deals with posture and body mechanics.

Most of the exercises in this chapter emphasize control of the tilt of the pelvis. This is because proper pelvic tilt improves posture and helps prevent back strain.

The more advanced exercises challenge abdominal muscles to work against the resistance of gravity, thereby improving the condition and strength of the muscular abdominal corset, and eventually leading to the acquisition of optimum abdominal power.

Note well
Exercises such as raising and lowering the trunk and the legs do involve leverage and force of gravity for resistance. The consensus of experts, however, is that these exercises are often ineffective for

strengthening the abdomen and are, in fact, potentially dangerous to the back. The actions involved in conventional sit-ups and double leg raising with legs straight depend largely on the flexor muscles of the hips, and not infrequently generate backache and back pain, because they exert undue pull on joints of the lumbar spine.

Before starting

Please *check with your doctor* before doing these or any other exercises.

Please warm up before practising the exercises (*see* chapter four).

A note to pregnant women

Except for the Abdominal Lift, the exercises in this chapter are safe for most pregnant women to practise, as long as the doctor approves, and provided they feel comfortable to do. However, I suggest a look at my book entitled *Easy Pregnancy with Yoga* (*see* Bibliography), which was written especially for the pre- and post-natal woman.

Hints on sit-up exercises

● Almost all the abdomen-strengthening effect of a sit-up occurs from the first 30 to 45 degrees; after that, the hip flexors take over. Simply curling up 17.5 to 20 centimetres (7 to 8 inches), keeping your waist on the surface on which you are exercising, is enough to exercise the abdominal muscles.

● The knees should be bent and the soles of the feet supported (for example, by the floor). This flattens and protects the lower back.

● The feet should *not* be held down. If they are, it could conceal weakness of the abdominals, while the hip flexors do the work.

● It is important to do diagonal movements

(such as the *Diagonal Curl-up*, Fig. 50), as well as straight up-and-down movements, to ensure exercise of all components of the muscular abdominal corset.

● Keep your chin tucked down; keep your back rounded rather than straight, since the latter promotes action of the hip flexors.

● Avoid jerking movements; curl up and down smoothly, in synchronization with regular breathing.

Preparing to exercise

Before practising the exercises to follow, be sure to warm up properly (*see* chapter four). Please also review the general instructions, also in chapter four which apply to the practice of all the exercises described in chapters five, six and seven. Here, for quick reference, is a summary of these instructions.

● Wear loose, comfortable clothing that permits you to breathe and stretch easily.

● Practise the exercises on a firm, padded surface, such as a carpeted floor (referred to as the 'mat').

● Concentration is essential: practise the exercises slowly and with complete awareness. Synchronize movement with regular breathing.

● Once you have completed the exercise, with no strain whatever, maintain the position for as many seconds as you wish, or can with absolute comfort (referred to as 'hold' the position).

● When holding the position, *do not* hold your breath; keep breathing naturally.

● When you are ready to come out of the position, do so slowly and with awareness; synchronize movement with regular breathing.

● After completing the exercise, rest briefly before practising another exercise.

At the end of your exercise session, cool down adequately (*see* chapter four for suggestions).

The Exercises

The Yoga Sit-up

1. Lie on your back, with your legs slightly apart and stretched out. Breathe regularly.

2. Bend your knees and slide your feet toward your buttocks, until the soles are flat on the mat. Maintain this distance between feet and buttocks while practising the exercise.

3. Rest the palms of your hands on your thighs.

4. Exhale as you slowly and carefully raise your head, keeping your gaze on your hands.

5. Reach for your knees, sliding your hands along the thighs, and keep your attention riveted on your hands, until you feel maximum tension in your abdominal muscles.

6. Hold this position for as long as you are comfortable in it (Fig. 48), but *do not* hold your breath. Keep breathing regularly.

7. Inhale and curl your spine onto the mat, resuming your starting position. Relax your arms and hands.

8. Rest briefly, breathing regularly.

Notes

● You may repeat the exercise once, and again later in the day.

● It is *not* necessary to touch the knees. Curl up only to the point where you feel maximum tightness of the abdominal muscles then stop there.

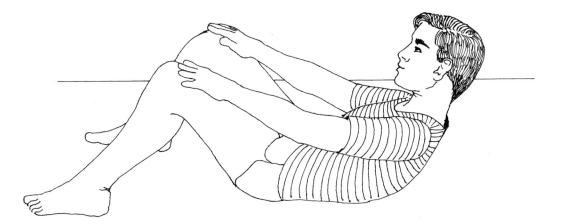

Fig. 48 Yoga Sit-up

The exercise to follow is advanced. Do it only if you feel ready for it. If you don't, proceed to the *Diagonal Curl-up* (Fig. 50).

The Angle Balance

1. Sit with your legs bent and the soles of your feet flat on the mat. Breathe regularly.

2. Tilt backward so that you balance on your bottom, bringing your legs closer to your body and your feet off the mat (use your hands to help, if necessary). Keep breathing regularly and concentrate on what you are doing. It will help you keep your balance.

3. Stretch out your arms so that they're parallel to the mat.

4. Attempt to straighten the legs; don't strain. It is not necessary for the legs to be straight, to begin with. When straightening them, you will need to adjust your degree of tilt to maintain your balance (Fig. 49).

5. Hold your balanced position for a few seconds to be begin with; longer as you become more comfortable in the position. Remember to breathe regularly.

6. Slowly and carefully resume your starting position.

7. Sit or lie down and rest.

8. Repeat the exercise once, if you wish. You may also repeat it later in the day.

Diagonal Curl-up

1. Lie on your back, with your knees bent and the soles of your feet flat on the mat. Keep your chin down, and breathe regularly.

2. Slowly, smoothly and carefully begin to

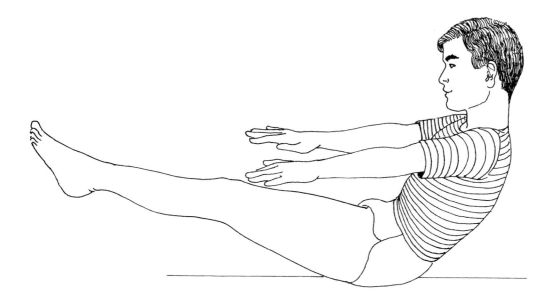

Fig. 49 Angle Balance

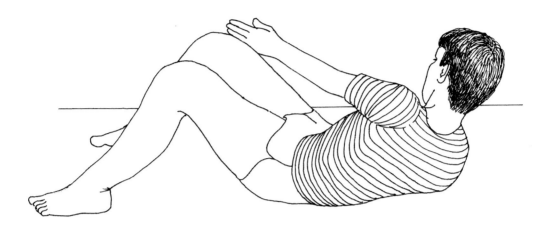

Fig. 50 Diagonal Curl-up

curl your body forward, reaching with your hands toward the outside of the *right* knee. Fix your attention on your hands (Fig. 50).

3. Hold this position for several seconds, or as long as you feel comfortable in it. *Do not* hold your breath; keep breathing regularly.

4. Slowly, smoothly and carefully roll back onto your mat, in reverse, to resume your starting position.

5. Stretch out and relax.

6. Repeat steps 2 to 4, this time reaching for the outside of the *left* knee.

7. Rest.

Advanced variation

As you acquire greater strength and become more confident, you may wish to try the Diagonal Curl-up with your arms folded across your chest or clasped behind your neck. In this case, aim your right shoulder toward your left knee as you curl forward, then repeat the curl up, aiming your left shoulder toward your right knee.

Single Leg Raise

1. Lie on your back, with your legs outstretched in front and your arms relaxed beside you. Breathe regularly.

2. Bend your *left* leg and rest the sole of the foot flat on the mat, a comfortable distance from your bottom.

3. On an *exhalation*, while pressing the small of the back firmly against the mat, slowly raise the straight leg until you feel the lower abdomen tighten. If you wish, you may aim your heel upward so as to benefit the hamstring muscles at the back of the leg (Fig. 51).

4. Hold the raised-leg position for a few seconds, or longer if you are comfortable doing so. *Do not* hold your breath; keep breathing regularly.

5. Keeping the small of the back firmly pressed to the mat, inhale and slowly lower your right leg to the mat.

6. Rest briefly before repeating the exercise with the same leg, if you wish.

7. Repeat steps 2 to 6, this time keeping the *right* leg bent, and raising the left leg.

Note well

Do *not* practise raising both legs together from a supine position. This exerts undue pull on spinal structures and puts the back at risk.

The Abdominal Lift

This is an advanced exercise. *Do not* practise it if you have high blood-pressure, an ulcer of the stomach or intestine (peptic ulcer), a heart problem or a hiatus hernia. Do *not*

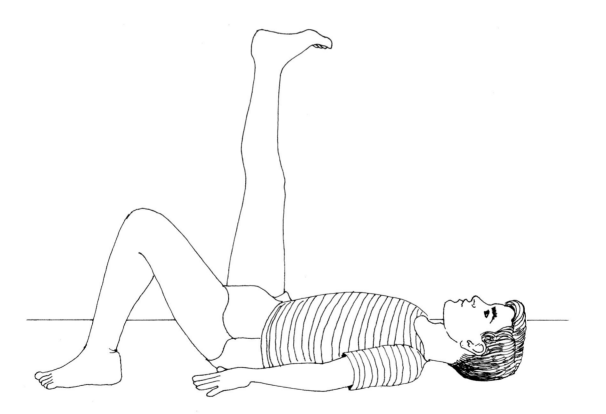

Fig. 51 Single Leg Raise

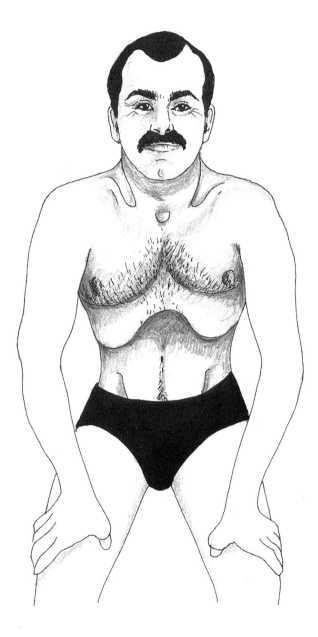

Fig. 52 *Abdominal Lift*

practise the *Abdominal Lift* if you are pregnant. In any case, do *check with your doctor* before attempting this exercise.

Practise the *Abdominal Lift* only on an empty or near-empty stomach; never immediately after having eaten.

1. Stand with your feet about 25 centimetres (10 inches) apart.

2. Bend your knees and turn them slightly outward, as if preparing to sit.

3. Place your hands on their respective

74

thighs. Keep your torso as erect as you comfortably can in this position. Breathe regularly.

4. E*xhale* and with the air still expelled, briskly *pull in your abdomen* as if to touch your spine with it, and *also pull it upward* toward your ribs (Fig. 52).

5. Hold the abdominal contraction until you feel the urge to inhale.

6. Inhale and straighten yourself. Rest briefly, resuming normal breathing.

7. Repeat the exercise once, if you wish. You may also repeat it later in the day.

To complete your abdominal exercises, please practise the Half Moon (Fig. 46) and the Spinal Twist (Fig. 47), both of which are described and illustrated in chapter five. These two exercises will condition your oblique abdominal muscles, part of the four-way abdominal corset described earlier in this chapter.

Cooling down

After your exercise session, do remember to cool down. Refer to chapter four for suggestions as to how to do so.

Chapter 7

Using the legs to spare the back

In chapter one, it was pointed out that certain leg muscles were considered secondary supports of the back, and that two of them contributed to the balance of the pelvic ring, thus helping maintain normal spinal curves. In chapter two, which dealt with posture and body mechanics, emphasis was placed on the use of the leg muscles to help prevent back strain.

It seems to make good sense, then, that if we're to 'use the legs to spare the back', the legs should be strong and flexible and functioning optimally. A brief look at the chief leg muscles involved in preventing backache therefore seems appropriate.

Leg muscles

Arising at the sides of the lumbar vertebrae, the *psoas* muscle passes along the groin and inserts into the upper thigh bone (femur). The *iliacus* arises from the hip bone and unites with the psoas to insert into the thigh as well. These two (ilio-psoas muscle) flex and rotate the thighs (hip flexors).

The *quadriceps* muscles, four altogether, are situated on the front of the thighs. They arise from the pelvis and the thigh bones and insert into the upper knee cap (patella). They extend, or straighten, the knees.

The *hamstrings*, of which there are three on each leg, run along the back of the thighs, passing from the lower pelvis to insert into the bones of the lower leg (tibia and fibula).

The *gluteal muscles*, forming the prominence of the buttocks, help raise the trunk from a stooping to an erect position and tighten the thighs and abduct them (move them away from the body).

Before starting the exercises
Please *check with your doctor* before doing these or any other exercises.

Pregnant women are referred to my book entitled *Easy Pregnancy with Yoga* (see bibliography).

Preparing to exercise

Before practising the exercises to follow, be sure to warm up properly (*see* chapter four). Please also review the general instructions, also in chapter four, which apply to the practice of all the exercises described in chapters five, six and seven. Here, for quick reference, is a summary of these instructions.

● Wear loose, comfortable clothing which permits you to breathe and stretch easily.

● Practise the exercises on a firm, padded surface, such as a carpeted floor (referred to as the 'mat').

● Concentrate fully on what you are doing. Synchronize your breathing with the body movements.

● Practise the exercises slowly and with complete awareness.

- Once you have completed the exercise, with no strain whatever, maintain the position for as many seconds as you wish or can with absolute comfort (referred to as 'hold' the position).

- When holding the position, *do not* hold your breath; keep breathing naturally.

- When you are ready to come out of the position, do so slowly and with awareness, your movements synchronized with your breathing.

- After completing the exercise, rest briefly before practising another exercise.

- At the end of your exercise session, cool down adequately (*see* chapter four for suggestions).

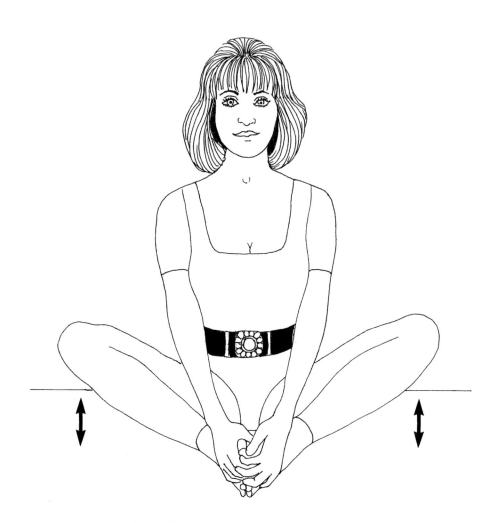

Fig. 53 *The Butterfly*

The Exercises

The Butterfly

1. Sit on your mat, with your legs folded inward and the soles of your feet together. Breathe regularly.

2. Carefully reach out and clasp your feet. If you can't, rest your hands on the mat beside you for support.

3. Keep breathing regularly as you move your knees down and up, at a slow to moderate pace. Do this several times (Fig. 53).

4. Place your hands on the mat (if you were holding your feet); tilt back slightly and stretch out your legs, one at a time.

5. Rest briefly, breathing regularly.

The Butterfly is an excellent warm-up for the legs and hip joints.

For additional exercise for the hip flexor muscles, please practise the knee presses (*see* chapter five).

Balance Posture

1. Stand tall, with your feet comfortably but not too far apart, and your body weight equally distributed. Breathe regularly.

2. Shift your weight onto your *right* foot. If you focus attention on your breathing, it will help you keep your balance.

3. Bend your *left* leg and point the foot backward; grasp the foot with the *left* hand, bringing it as close to the buttock as you can with absolute comfort.

4. Keep breathing regularly as you raise your *right* arm upward, to help maintain balance. Keep your torso as erect as possible (Fig. 54).

5. Hold the position as long as you wish to or can, remembering to breathe regularly

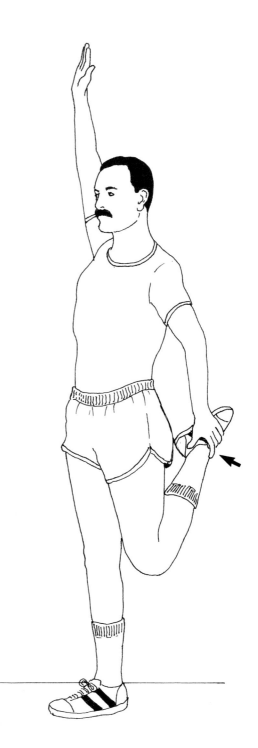

Fig. 54 *Balance Posture*

79

and to focus attention on the flow of the breath to help keep you steady.

6. Slowly resume your starting position. Rest briefly.

7. Repeat steps 2 to 6, this time balancing on the *left* foot. Relax at the end of the exercise.

The Balance Posture, sometimes referred to as 'The Quadriceps Stretch', conditions the quadriceps muscles, as the name suggests. It also develops and enhances concentration which, experts say, is a prerequisite for activities such as lifting safely (*see* chapter two).

I sometimes practise a lying version of the Balance Posture, thus:

1. Lie prone (face downward), then turn your head to one side for ease of breathing. You may place a flat cushion or folded towel (or even your hands) under your pelvis to reduce the arch of your lower back. Keep your legs close together or comfortably separated.

2. Keep breathing regularly and bend your legs, bringing the heels toward the buttocks. You should feel a delightful, therapeutic stretch of the thigh muscles as you do so.

3. You may alternately bend and straighten the legs, at a slow pace, several times in succession; or you may bend them, hold the position as long as you're comfortable doing so, then rest. Keep breathing regularly throughout the exercise, and rest briefly afterwards.

Easy variation

For those of you who find it difficult to do the Balance Posture without the aid of a prop, you may hold on with one hand to something stable (such as a post or a sturdy piece of furniture), using the free hand to grasp the foot, as described in step 3 of the basic exercise.

The Dog Stretch

1. Start in an 'all-fours' position, on hands and knees. Your thighs should be roughly perpendicular to the mat and your arms sloping gently forward.

2. Tuck your toes forward; rock back slightly; raise your knees and straighten your legs; straighten your arms; look downward. You're now in a hips-high, head-low position (*see* Fig. 31, chapter four). Keep breathing regularly. Slowly and carefully and with full attention, aim your heels toward the mat until you feel a pleasant stretch of the muscles along the back of your legs (the hamstrings). At the first hint of discomfort, stop and slowly resume your starting position. Otherwise, hold the position for several seconds or as long as you are comfortable in it, breathing regularly all the while.

3. Slowly and carefully rock forward and resume your beginning position, on all-fours.

4. Sit on your heels, Japanese style (*see* chapter two, Fig. 9).

5. Now go into the *Pose of a Child* (*see* chapter five, Fig. 45), or a variation of that position, in which you keep your arms stretched out ahead of you. Relax for a while, breathing regularly. With each exhalation, let go of any residual tension you may be feeling.

Other exercises beneficial to the hamstring muscles include lunging (*see* chapter two, Fig. 19), the Rock-and-roll (*see* chapter four, Fig. 23) and ankle rotation (*see also* chapter four).

The Half Locust

1. Lie on your abdomen, with your chin touching the mat and your legs fairly close together. Straighten your arms and position them, close together, under your body. Make fists and keep the thumbs

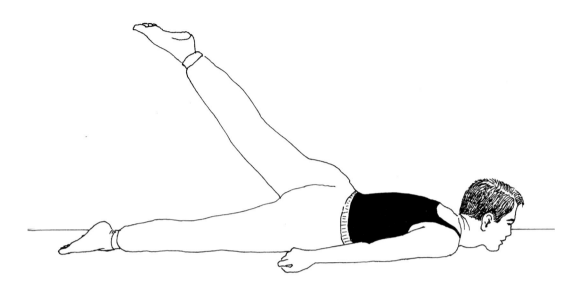

Fig. 55 Half Locust

down. (You may, alternatively, keep your arms alongside your body.) Breathe regularly.

2. E*xhale* and slowly and carefully raise one still-straight leg as high as you comfortably can, while keeping your chin, arms and body pressed to the mat (Fig. 55).

3. Hold the raised-leg posture as long as you comfortably can, breathing regularly as you do so.

4. Slowly and carefully lower your leg. Rest briefly. Continue breathing regularly.

5. Repeat the exercise with the other leg.

Following practice of the Half Locust, you may try resting in the Pose of a Child position (*see* chapter five, Fig. 45).

Toe-finger Posture (Standing)

1. Stand naturally erect, with your body weight equally distributed between your feet, and your hands relaxed at your sides. Breathe regularly.

2. Shift your weight onto one foot. Exhaling, *carefully* raise the other foot off the mat, bending the leg and bringing the foot toward you.

3. Grasp the toes of the raised foot with one or both hands. (If using one hand, swing the other hand to the side to help you maintain balance.) Keep breathing regularly, and focus attention on your breathing, which also helps you keep balance.

4. Keeping a firm grasp on the toes, *carefully* try to straighten the raised leg, alert for any hint of strain on the hamstring muscles, at the back of the leg (Fig. 56).

5. Hold the position as long as you can maintain balance, breathing regularly.

6. Bend the raised leg, release the grasp on

81

the toes and resume your starting position (as in step 1).

7. Rest briefly.

8. Repeat the exercise, this time standing on the other foot.

9. You may repeat the entire exercise once now and once again later in the day.

The Toe-finger Posture (Standing) is not only excellent for improving the tone of the hamstring muscles at the back of the legs, but also for strengthening the ankles and the abdomen. It is, in addition, superb for developing concentration, which is a prerequisite for the safe performance of activities such as bending, getting up, lifting and shovelling (*see* chapter 2).

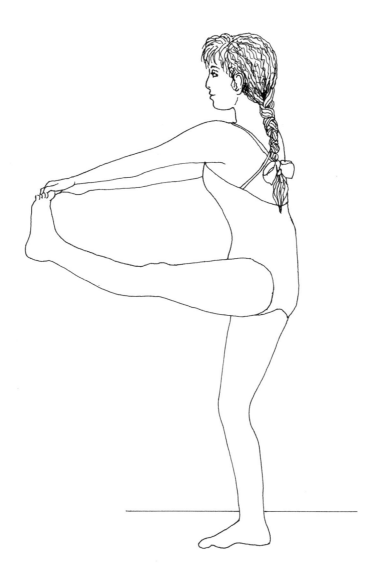

Fig. 56 Toe-finger Posture (Standing)

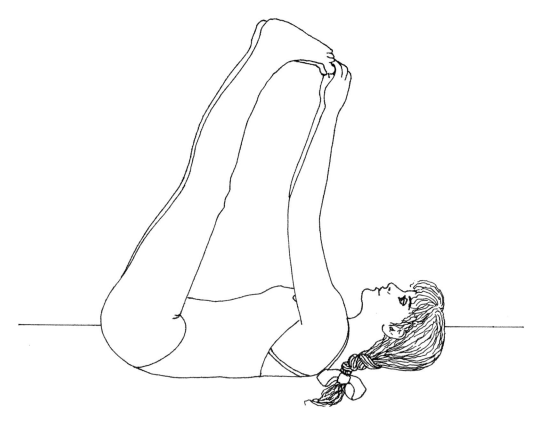

Fig. 57 *Toe-finger Posture (Supine)*

Variation

The following is a challenging variation to the Toe-finger Posture (Standing). In addition to the benefits mentioned, this variation also conditions the inner leg muscles.

1. Begin as in step 1 of the basic exercise, just described.

2. Shift your weight onto one foot.

3. Raise the other foot and grasp the toes with *one hand* only. Swing the other hand sideways to help you maintain balance.

4. *Carefully* attempt to straighten the raised leg. Remember to breathe regularly to help you keep your balance.

5. *Slowly*, and with control, bring the raised leg to the side, as far as you comfortably can.

6. Hold the position as long as you can maintain balance, breathing regularly.

7. *Slowly* bring the raised leg back to the front.

8. *Carefully* resume your starting position.

9. Rest briefly.

10. Repeat the exercise with the other leg.

11. Rest.

Toe-finger Posture (Supine)

This is a favourite of mine, which I find marvellous for helping relieve a tired back.

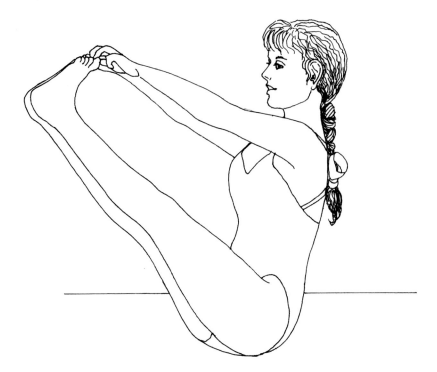

Fig. 58   *Toe-finger Posture (Sitting)*

It is also wonderful for conditioning the hamstring and other leg muscles.

1. Lie on your back (supine), with your legs stretched out in front of you and your arms relaxed at your sides. Breathe regularly.

2. Bend first one leg and then the other, bringing the soles of your feet flat on the mat.

3. Bring one bent knee and then the other toward your chest.

4. Tuck the fingers of the left hand under the toes of the left foot; do the same with the other fingers and toes.

5. Holding the toes securely, *slowly and carefully* straighten your legs (Fig. 57). Do *not strain*. As you become more flexible, it will be easier to achieve the posture in the illustration.

6. Hold the position as long as you wish to, or can with absolute comfort. Do *not* hold your breath. Keep breathing regularly.

7. Bend your legs and, one at a time, put the soles of your feet flat on the mat before resuming your starting position ~ (as in step 1).

8. Rest.

Variation

1. Begin as in step 1 of the basic exercise.

2. Proceed to steps 2, 3 and 4 of the basic exercise.

3. When you have assumed the position depicted in Fig. 57, maintain a firm hold on the toes and *slowly and carefully* spread your legs apart to their comfortable limit.

4. Hold the spread-leg position as long as

you can with absolute comfort. Keep breathing regularly.

5. Slowly bring your legs together (Fig. 57).

6. Bend your legs and, one at a time, put the soles of your feet flat on the mat before resuming your starting position.

7. Rest.

Toe-finger Posture (Sitting)

This posture is reminiscent of the Angle Balance (*see* chapter six, Fig. 49) and, like it, is an exercise in concentration.

The Toe-finger Posture (Sitting) has the additional advantage of conditioning the leg muscles, especially the hamstring and the quadriceps, so important in helping maintain good balance of the pelvic ring, and consequently good posture (*see* chapter one).

1. Sit with your legs bent and your soles flat on the mat. Breathe regularly.

2. Bring your knees close to your chest, at the same time tilting backward so that you are balancing on your bottom, with your feet lifted off the mat.

3. Reach out and firmly tuck the fingers of your left hand under the toes of the left foot; do the same with the right fingers and toes. Keep breathing regularly to help you maintain your balance.

4. Keeping a firm hold on the toes, *slowly and carefully* begin to straighten your legs without losing balance (Fig. 58).

5. Hold the position as long as you comfortably can.

6. Release the hold on the toes, bring the knees toward the chest and resume your starting position, as in step 1.

7. Rest.

Cooling down

After completing your exercise session, do remember to cool down. Refer to chapter four for suggestions as to how to do so.

Chapter 8

Relaxing for a pain-free back

No one can say with certainty why some individuals are more susceptible to back pain than others of similar build and lifestyle. But experts believe that the answer lies partly in the psyche. They base this belief on the observation that suppressed emotions are often at the root of muscular tension which generates pain in the back and head and elsewhere in the body. In short, physical symptoms can be symbolic of underlying psychological problems.

Those who are sceptical of this have only to consider such common reactions as blushing because of embarrassment, and sexual arousal at the mere thought of an object of attraction. The mechanisms responsible for these responses may be similar to those producing backache. Indeed, there are many case histories written to illustrate that backache and back pain stem from sources of distress buried in the deep recesses of the mind. One such case is cited by Kenneth Pelletier who tells of a middle-aged cardiologist (heart specialist) with a chronic back problem. His doctor discovered, during therapy, that when the patient was a teenager, he had received a blow from his father. Knocked down windless, the boy huffed and puffed and arched his shoulders backward, desperately trying to get his wind back. Subsequently, whenever under intense stress, the cardiologist would automatically repeat the rapid breathing and the arching of the back which had brought him relief when he was struck as a boy. Unfortunately, these strategies only aggravated his back problem as an adult.

The states of our mind are a reflection of the states of our back and, though the back is behind us, it rules our every mood (Leboyer, 21).

Understanding Pain

The degree of pain experienced is influenced not only by physical factors (such as pressure on nerve endings), but also by religious beliefs, ethnicity and personality. Also playing a part in how we respond to pain stimuli are memory, attention, fear, depression and causes of stress such as job dissatisfaction. All these can intensify and prolong backache and back pain.

Tolerating Pain

In the 1960s, Ronald Melzack, a professor at McGill University, Canada, and Patrick Wall, proposed a theory as to why some individuals seem to tolerate pain better than others. They put forth a spinal 'gate control theory' in which they suggested the existence of a nervous mechanism that, in effect, opens or closes a 'gate' regulating the pain stimuli that reach the brain for interpretation. This mechanism can be affected by certain psychological processes, such as those mentioned earlier: fear, cultural heritage and personality components.

Steven Brena, MD, author of *Yoga & Medicine*, gives an example of how the spinal gate mechanism probably works. Imagine standing in a field or campsite, holding a paper cup of hot beverage. You spill some and burn yourself. You drop the cup and shake your hand around. Now visualize being in your employer's home. In your hand you hold an expensive china cup of tea. Again you burn yourself. This time, however, *you first put the cup down safely, then you shake your hand.* Why are there two different reactions to similar incidents? In the second example, when the sensation of burning was relayed to the brain, you very quickly *evaluated* the consequences of damaging your employer's rug or breaking the china teacup. The emotional centres in your brain inhibited further sensations of pain until *after* you safely put down the cup and avoided soiling the rug. In the first example, no such inhibition occurred because, upon assessment, you determined that no harm could come to the field or to the paper cup you let fall.

The foregoing is in accord with the spinal gate control theory. Simply put, when the gate is 'open', painful impulses can get through to the brain where they are interpreted as pain. When the gate is 'closed', however, few or no sensations get through. The spinal gate shuts out, as it were, the entry of sensory inputs.

Closing the gate

How can we close our spinal gate to prevent some of the painful stimuli from reaching the brain? How can we alter our mental evaluation of the hurt?

We can use drugs, such as pain relievers and tranquillizers, to dull emotional responses. These medications, however, can produce side effects such as nausea, high or low blood pressure, dizziness, headache, constipation and other unpleasant symptoms. Alternatively, we can use natural pain control measures.

Natural pain control

According to Dr Brena, everyone has the capacity for limiting or even preventing pain through will-power. Natural pain control methods are largely based on 'closing the gate' to the entry of pain stimuli. Compared with drugs, natural methods have the advantage of producing no deleterious effects. What they do is mobilize the body's own resources to regulate pain and promote well-being. Currently used methods of pain relief include acupuncture, TENS (Transcutaneous Electrical Nerve Stimulation), psychotherapy, biofeedback, hypnosis, the application of heat or cold and massage. These are well-respected, effective pain control approaches. They do, however, require the help of an outside agent, such as a therapist or a machine or gadget. With yoga techniques, however, you rely entirely on your own natural resources, which are with you wherever you may be.

Note well
If your pain persists, be sure to see a doctor.

Pain relief through yoga

Yoga pain relief techniques work on the following principles:

● trying to prevent painful impulses at the periphery (extremities of the body);

● trying to stop painful impulses as they travel along the spinal cord;

● altering or reducing the perception of, and reaction to, the pain;

● encouraging a greater amount of oxygen to reach body tissues and wash away irritants, and

- attempting to re-educate disused muscles.

The techniques that follow work on these principles.

Meditation

Briefly defined, meditation is doing one thing and only one thing at a tirne. You focus your attention on one object or activity at a time to the exclusion of everything else.

Chief among the many benefits derived from regular meditation are: the ability to relax while maintaining mental alertness, and increased skin resistance which indicates decreased tension and anxiety.

More and more, doctors are recommending a period of daily meditation for various health disorders. For your own reassurance, however, *do obtain your doctor's permission* to practise the specimen meditations that follow.

Before starting your meditation

- select a reasonably quiet place where you won't be interrupted for about half an hour;

- sit comfortably, on a mat or in a chair which adequately supports your spine;

- maintain a well-aligned spinal column and a relaxed body (regular practice of a relaxation technique, such as the Toe-to-top exercise in chapter four, Fig. 33, will train you to achieve a high degree of relaxation in a short time);

- establish a slow, quiet, regular breathing rhythm, through the nostrils, and

- be completely aware of what you are doing.

Having met all these requirements, you are now ready to begin. Do not be discouraged

if you find your mind wandering at first. With regular practice, this will occur less and less, so do persevere.

A Basic Meditation

1. Sit comfortably with your body relaxed. Pay special attention to your jaws; unclench your teeth and keep your lips together but not compressed. Rest your hands quietly in your lap, on your knees or on an armrest.

2. Close your eyes.

3. Breathe regularly.

4. On an *exhalation*, mentally say the word 'one'.

5. Inhale.

6. Repeat steps 4 and 5 again and again in slow, smooth succession, always silently saying 'one' on the *exhalation*.

Whenever your attention strays from your meditation, gently guide it back and start again at step 4.

Instead of the word 'one', you may use any monosyllable or short phrase, such as 'peace', 'love and peace', 'relax' or 'be calm'.

When you feel the need to end your meditation, open your eyes, slowly stretch your limbs or massage them, or do gentle warm-ups as described in chapter four. Take your time getting up. Never rush.

A healing meditation

1. Sit comfortably with your body relaxed. Pay special attention to your jaws; unclench your teeth and keep your lips together but not compressed. Rest your hands quietly in your lap, on your knees or on an armrest.

2. Close your eyes.

3. Breathe regularly.

4. As you inhale, visualize an intake of healing energy: silently tell yourself: 'I'm breathing in healing energy', focusing attention on the part of your body that is uncomfortable. You could, for example, picture this healing energy as a beam of gentle light penetrating your body, along with the incoming breath, reaching the affected part, bringing it warmth and comfort.

5. As you exhale, visualize the elimination of pain-producing substances: silently tell yourself, 'I'm breathing out harmful substances', again focusing attention on the affected body part. You could, for instance, imagine these substances as a stream of toxic wastes flowing from the body, with the outgoing breath, and emptying into a dark river, never to return.

6. Repeat the process, as in steps 4 and 5, again and again, in slow, smooth succession, for the predetermined length of your meditation (usually twenty minutes, although you could start with ten).

Whenever your attention strays from your meditation, gently guide it back and start again at step 4.

When you feel the need to end your meditation, open your eyes, slowly stretch your limbs or massage them, or do gentle warm-ups as described in chapter 4. Take your time getting up. Never rush.

Variations on a healing meditation

1. Follow steps 1 to 3 of the healing meditation just described.

2. If practicable, rest your hands lightly on or over the affected body part, having first warmed them by rubbing them briskly together several times.

3. As you inhale, visualize a warm, soothing stream of water trickling along your arms, through your fingers and onto the part that hurts, gently and lovingly bathing it.

4. As you exhale, visualize the hurt or pain – in the form of a mist perhaps – drifting away on the outgoing breath and dissipating into the atmosphere.

5. Repeat steps 3 and 4 again and again, in smooth succession, as long as you wish or can, or until you experience relief.

If your attention wanders, simply redirect it to your meditation and start again.

Remember to come out of your meditation slowly and with awareness, as described in the basic meditation.

Here are other suggested forms of visualization to try:

● With your mind's eye, picture a soft brush dusting away powder-like deposits that have settled around the joints of your vertebral column, making them stiff and painful. Synchronize the 'brushing' with each inhalation; with each exhalation, imagine the deposits floating away and scattering into the air, never to return.

● Visualize gentle, loving hands applying a soothing, healing balm to the skin over the affected part. As the balm is absorbed through the skin, visualize the affected part becoming less tense, more relaxed, and the hurt disappearing. Synchronize these visualizations with your breathing, which should always be slow and smooth.

● Imagine listening to the dulcet tones of distant music. Feel it at work assuaging your anguish and bringing you comfort.

There are infinite possibilities. The imagery you select should reflect your own natural inclinations and you should be comfortable with it.

Ending the meditation

Never get up suddenly after your meditation. Open your eyes and sit quietly for a minute or two until you've become accustomed to the light. Practise gentle warm-up exercises such as moving your fingers and toes about, rotating your ankles, head and shoulders or leisurely stretching your limbs. Take a few slow, smooth, deep breaths. Get up carefully.

Concentration

Concentration, observed the late psychoanalyst Dr Erich Fromm in his well-known work *The Art of Loving*, is rare in our culture. We're inclined to do several things at once: read, listen to the radio or talk while smoking, eating and/or drinking. Yet in order to prevent injury and to be successful in whatever we set out to do, we need to know how to direct and hold attention on one thing or person at a time, regardless of distracting stimuli.

Because of this predisposition for doing several things at once, we often find it difficult to be still. Observe those in any group of which you are a part and you will note how few hands and mouths are at rest. It seems that there is always a compulsion to talk and to move about.

It is only when we learn to be physically and mentally still, however, that we can hope to master the art of concentration. For it is only then that we can give to an activity that undivided attention that is necessary for promoting safety and effectiveness.

It is a misconception that concentrating on something depletes our energy and generates fatigue. When we focus attention on one thing to the exclusion of everything else, it in fact promotes alertness, and the tiredness that follows is healthful rather than enervating.

Since no art can be learned, let alone mastered, without regular practice, here are simple, effective concentration techniques for you to try as part of your daily exercise programme. (The Angle Balance, the Balance Posture, and the Toe-finger Posture, standing and sitting, as depicted by Figs. 49, 54, 56 and 58, also help develop concentration.)

To prepare for the concentration techniques, follow the instructions given earlier in this chapter as prerequisites for meditation.

Candle concentration

For this exercise, place a lighted candle at or slightly below eye level, on a table or stool, depending on where you are sitting.

1. Look intently at the candle flame, remembering to maintain regular breathing (Fig. 59). If you need to blink, do so.

2. Now close your eyes and retain or recall the image of the flame. If it disappears, don't be anxious. Mentally gaze in the direction of its disappearance and persuade it to come back. Keep breathing regularly.

3. After two minutes, open your eyes. Relax.

With each subsequent exercise session, increase the time spent looking at the flame itself, and that spent recalling its image, until your exercise lasts from five to ten minutes.

Variation

Instead of a candle, you may use any other small, pleasing object, such as a flower, a fruit, a design or even a stone on the beach.

Respiratory Concentration

1. Sit comfortably. Relax your body. Breathe regularly. Close your eyes.

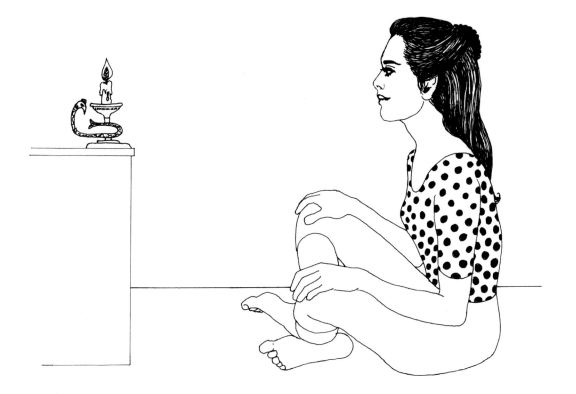

Fig. 59 Candle Concentration

2. Inhale and mentally count 'one thousand, two thousand, three thousand . . .', and so on, until your inhalation is complete.

3. Exhale and mentally count as in step 2. Lessen or increase your count to match the length of your respirations.

4. Repeat smooth, steady inhalations and exhalations through the nostrils, in synchronization with your silent counting, for about two minutes to begin with, working up to about ten minutes as you progress in your practice.

If your mind strays from the breathing and the counting, gently guide it back and resume this rhythmic exercise.

Concentration on sound

1. Sit comfortably. Check that your jaws are not tight (unclench your teeth) and your lips not compressed (they should touch each other lightly). Relax the rest of your body. Breathe regularly. Close your eyes.

2. On your next *exhalation*, say 'Hmmm . . .', until your exhalation is complete.

3. Inhale silently through the nostrils.

4. Repeat steps 2 and 3, humming on the exhalation and inhaling without humming.

Practise this exercise for about two minutes to begin with, working up to about five minutes as you become more comfortable with the technique.

Try to become totally absorbed in the sound. If your attention drifts, coax it back to concentration on the breathing and on the humming.

Breathing Exercises

Earlier in this chapter, I outlined principles on which yoga pain-relief techniques work. The visualization exercises described are useful in helping alter or reduce the perception of, and reaction to, any discomfort or pain felt. They help prevent painful stimuli from reaching the brain.

The breathing exercises which follow are also based on these principles. In addition, they encourage a better oxygen supply to reach body tissues to wash away irritants contributing to discomfort and pain. They also help reeducate the muscles involved in the breathing process, chiefly the diaphragm, which is situated between the chest and the abdomen.

Prerequisites for effective breathing

1. A naturally erect position of the vertebral column (spine), with the ribcage relaxed so as to avoid compression of the lungs and other major organs in the chest (heart and large blood vessels).

2. A slow, steady, deep inhalation, first using the diaphragm somewhat as a suction pump, and then expanding the ribcage with the help of the chest muscles (Brena, 90).

3. A slow, steady exhalation, using mainly the diaphragm in reverse action as a sort of a squeezing pump.

4. A regular breathing rhythm.

5. Unless otherwise specified, breathing through the nostrils, with the mouth closed, so that the air may be warmed and filtered before reaching the lungs.

6. A relaxed body (pay special attention to the jaws, face and hands).

After breathing slowly and deeply, the oxygenation of the blood is known to improve. This means better nourishment of body tissues, and improved elimination of waste products injurious to health.

Supine Abdominal Breathing

1. Lie on your back, with your legs outstretched in front and comfortably separated. Bend your arms and rest the palms of your hands flat on your abdomen so that the tips of the middle fingers meet above your navel. Close your eyes.

2. Begin with a slow, smooth inhalation through the nostrils, making it as deep as possible without incurring discomfort. Focus your attention on the muscular movements of your chest and abdomen: your ribcage expands and your abdomen rises. The fingers separate.

3. Exhale slowly and smoothly through the nostrils, again focusing attention on the chest and abdomen: the ribcage relaxes and the abdomen flattens. The middle fingers again touch in midline.

4. Repeat steps 2 and 3 in smooth succession for several minutes.

5. Relax your arms and hands at your sides. Breathe regularly.

Variation

Instead of having your legs stretched out in front, you may bend them, placing the feet flat on the surface on which you are lying, a comfortable distance from your bottom. I like positioning my legs so that my knees lean against each other and my feet are apart.

A dynamic cleansing breath

In addition to being an excellent breathing exercise, this dynamic cleansing breath (sometimes called the 'pumping breath') is superb for helping firm the abdominal muscles. Please review chapter six in connection with the importance of good abdominal muscle tone for the general health of the back.

Stage I

1. Lie on your back, with your legs stretched out in front and comfortably separated. Rest your arms beside you. Keep your head, neck, shoulders, arms and legs relaxed. Close your eyes. Breathe regularly through your nostrils. Focus your attention on your abdomen.

2. Inhale steadily and deeply through your nostrils so that your abdomen swells out.

3. Without pausing, briskly expel the air from your lungs (your abdomen will flatten and tighten).

4. Inhalation will follow, almost involuntarily.

5. Continue regular breathing.

Stage II

Now that you have experienced the action involved in this dynamic breathing exercise, you may proceed to stage II, as follows:

● Practise steps 2 and 3 above, several times in succession (ten times if you can).

● Rest afterwards, breathing regularly.

Variation

You may practise the dynamic cleansing breath while sitting or standing.

Note well

This is a fairly powerful breathing technique which is *not* recommended for pregnant women.

If you suffer from any circulatory or breathing problems, do first *check with your doctor* before trying this breathing exercise.

The Alternate Nostril Breath

Here is a very soothing breathing exercise. It helps alleviate anxiety, which worsens physical discomforts and pain. It is also a useful antidote for sleeplessness, which is a problem for many back sufferers.

1. Sit with your spine held naturally erect, or properly supported. Relax your body, making a quick top-to-toe check. Relax your jaws. Breathe regularly through your nostrils.

2. Rest your left hand quietly in your lap, on your knee or on an armrest.

3. Arrange the fingers of your *right* hand as depicted in the illustration (Fig. 60): the right thumb is used to close the right nostril; the two middle fingers are curled toward the palm, and the ring and little fingers are used to close the left nostril. (If you find the foregoing awkward, you may rest the two middle fingers lightly above the bridge of the nose once the breathing exercise is in progress.)

4. Close your eyes and begin: close your right nostril and inhale slowly, smoothly and deeply through the left nostril.

5. Close your left nostril and release closure of the right; exhale.

6. Inhale through the right nostril.

7. Close the right nostril; release closure of the left nostril and exhale.

Relaxing for a pain-free back

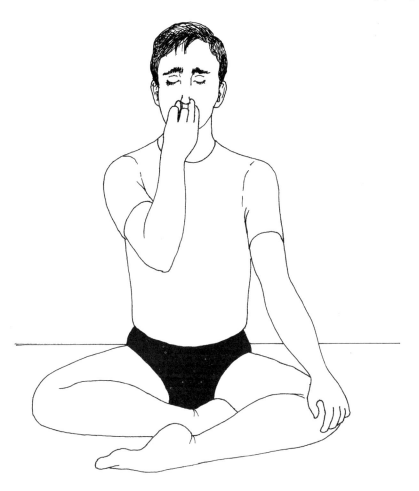

Fig. 60 The Alternate Nostril Breath

This completes one round of alternate nostril breathing.

8. Repeat steps 4 to 7 in smooth succession, as many times as you wish, until you feel a sense of calm and well-being.

9. Relax your right arm. Resume regular breathing. Open your eyes.

All-body Relaxation

The following exercise is a variation of the Toe-to-top relaxation (Savasana), illustrated in Fig. 33, chapter four. In this exercise, however, you dispense with the tensing of muscle groups prior to relaxing them. As well, you can practise this all-body relaxation technique in a variety of places: on your exercise mat; in an easy chair, on your bed or even sitting upright in your doctor's waiting-room. Close your eyes or keep them open, as circumstances permit.

Here's how to do it:

1. Start with your feet, isolating them, as it were, from the rest of your body. Give

95

them silent suggestion to let go of tightness; to relax. For instance you may, in your mind, say: 'Toes relax. Feet relax.' Consciously let go of the tension you feel in them. Be aware that they are becoming more relaxed than before. Keep breathing regularly.

2. Next, focus attention on your lower legs. Again, give silent suggestion to them to let go of tension; to relax. Concentrate on the calf muscles; try to be aware of the tightness in them disappearing.

3. Move upward to the thigh muscles (the quadriceps). Give the same positive mental suggestion to let go of tightness; to relax.

4. Next, give attention to the abdominal muscles: as you breathe in, be aware of the abdomen rising and as you breathe out note how it falls and relaxes. Do this a few times.

5. Continue in this manner, isolating various body parts, concentrating on each in turn while giving silent suggestion to let go of tightness; to relax. The following sequence is suggested:

   Move from the abdomen to the ribcage; synchronize your breathing with the movement of the chest. Inhale and note how the chest expands; exhale and note how it relaxes.

   Proceed to the back of the body: the buttocks and lower back; the small of the back, at waist level; the upper back, between the shoulderblades.

   Attend next to the hands, arms and shoulders. Follow this with the elimination of tension from the neck.

   Finish with the facial and scalp muscles: the jaws, lips, tongue, cheeks, eyes, forehead and scalp.

6. End with full attention to your breathing. Each time you inhale, visualize an intake of good things: of health, of freedom from discomfort, of energy; whatever you find easiest to picture. Each time you exhale, visualize an outflow of everything unwanted: toxins, ill feelings, pain; whatever you find convenient to imagine. Also, with each exhalation, let yourself sink more deeply into the surface on which you are lying or sitting, increasingly relaxed. Surrender yourself completely to the sensation of calm that enfolds you.

Remember to come out of your state of relaxation slowly. Take your time, moving your fingers and toes, rolling your head from side to side, or gently stretching your limbs. Remember also to get up carefully.

Sleeping for Backache Relief

Every year, tons of sleeping pills are consumed by thousands of individuals seeking relief from the inability to enjoy a good night's sleep. Why is it that some people seem to function well with a mere four hours of sleep, while others wake up tired and aching after eight hours in bed?

The causes of insomnia, or habitual sleeplessness, fall roughly under two headings: non-physical causes, as seen in anxiety states, and physical, as in bodily discomfort or pain, such as backache. Often, however, people say they have insomnia because of a long-term dissatisfaction with the duration and/or the quality of sleep. Some individuals become obsessed with the idea that they must have eight hours of sleep each night. If they miss a half-hour, they view it as a disaster. The fact is that some people need only five or six hours' sleep at night to function optimally the next day. Moreover, as we grow older, we tend to need less sleep than when we were younger.

The first remedy for sleeplessness is to determine the cause or causes of it. Here are fourteen questions to ask yourself to help you pinpoint what's at the root of your inability to have a restful night's sleep.

1. What causes you to awaken during the night (for example, pain, hunger, having to go to the toilet)?

2. Is your insomnia a possible side effect of medication you are taking?

3. Do you take a nap in the evening after supper?

4. Do you habitually drink alcoholic beverages in the evening to help you fall asleep?

5. Do you drink tea, coffee or other beverages containing caffeine before going to sleep?

6. Do you eat a large meal shortly before going to sleep?

7. Do you smoke before going to sleep?

8. Do you exercise vigorously before going to sleep?

9. Do you take a *hot* shower or bath before going to bed for the night?

10. Do you read exciting stories or watch stimulating television shows before going to bed?

11. Are your bed and bedclothes absolutely comfortable?

12. Is your room temperature too hot or too cold?

13. Do you often go to bed with unresolved problems on your mind?

14. Have you discussed your sleep problem with a health professional?

The answers to the foregoing questions should enable you to gain some insight into why you are not enjoying a refreshing night's sleep. A checkup with your doctor is also a good idea, to help rule out any physical causes at the root of the problem.

Remedies for sleeplessness

Orthodox medical treatments for insomnia and other forms of sleeplessness rely heavily on medications. These drugs, however, are not without unpleasant side effects. Certain hypnotic agents can, in fact, disturb the normal sleep cycle and produce drowsiness, confusion and memory loss. Long-term use of pharmaceutical sleep aids simply mask the problem; they do not solve it.

The following, by contrast, are natural measures to promote sound sleep. They do not produce the adverse reactions some drugs do.

Sleep serves two primary functions: to restore energy and to help the body regulate and synchronize itself. Studies show that people deprived of sleep show various adverse symptoms, including psychotic behaviour.

With specific reference to the health of the spine, I mentioned in chapter one that when we are sleeping or resting, the intervertebral discs suck in water and other nutrients. This compensates for the squeezing out of fluids from the discs when we are awake and active.

Recipe for a good night's sleep

The following are some of the main ingredients necessary for a night of sound, refreshing sleep.

Pre-sleep activities

Mild exercise after supper can promote sound sleep, whereas vigorous exercise may prove too stimulating. All the exercises in chapter four are suitable to practise at night before going to sleep. The breathing exercises are also appropriate, as well as the all-body relaxation technique described in this chapter.

A warm (*not* hot) bath is relaxing, and some people find it sleep-inducing. The water should be between 35°C and 38°C (95°F –

100°F). *See also* the section on herbal baths later in this chapter.

It is not a good idea to take a nap in the evening, as it may interfere with your night's sleep.

Avoid reading stimulating literature or watching disturbing television shows if you have observed that they detract from the quality of your night's sleep.

As you prepare to sleep, try to turn your thoughts away from unpleasant matters. Consciously try to focus attention on positive experiences instead. Practise the Toe-to-top relaxation exercise described in chapter four, and toward the end of it spend a few minutes visualizing a peaceful scene or recalling an experience that brought you joy and contentment. You may also practise the Supine Abdominal Breathing exercise or the Alternate Nostril Breath following the Toe-to-top relaxation.

Food, drink and tobacco

Make your last meal of the day a light and easily digested one. If you find that you can't sleep because you are hungry, place a light snack at your bedside, such as cereal or a thermos of warm milk, so you don't have to go to the kitchen to prepare it. (The calcium in the milk, in addition to being sleep promoting, is good for your bones, and the amino acid tryptophan, which it also contains, is a known soporific.) Two or three calcium tablets taken with the warm milk is another good relaxant, especially if you have a calcium deficiency. *Check with your doctor or nutrition counsellor.*

Avoid drinking alcoholic beverages shortly before bedtime, since they detract from the quality of sleep. Also, avoid stimulants such as tea, coffee, cocoa and cola drinks at night.

Heating, ventilation, noise and light

Before going to bed for the night, check that the room temperature is comfortable. Some people find that a somewhat cool temperature is more conducive to restful slumber than one which is too warm.

If the room is stuffy, it may cause you to wake up in the morning feeling less than refreshed. If the weather is suitable, try sleeping with a window open.

Heavy curtains help to darken a room and keep out disturbing sounds. Ticking clocks should be removed if they bother you, and rattling doors and windows should be fixed.

Bed and bedding

The bed on which you habitually sleep should be sufficiently firm to give your body good support without causing stiffness, aches or other forms of discomfort. If your mattress sags, it will subject major muscles and ligaments to strain and produce tension buildup.

Whereas some people are high in their praise of waterbeds, others are sceptical of them. Do experiment to find out what is best for *you*.

If you have neck problems, consider using an improvised neck collar: roll a small towel into a sausage shape, and place it around your neck. This will give your neck support and prevent your head from rolling.

Keep bedclothes to a minimum. Heavy bedding may impede the proper circulation of blood.

Some individuals find that the position of the bed makes a difference to the quality of their sleep. Sleeping in a north-to-south position, they find, is more conducive to restful slumber and a feeling of vitality next day than when they sleep in an east-to-west position. This is probably because the body, being a magnetic field, better harmonizes with the earth's magnetic current when placed in the former position.

If you are very sensitive and suffer from insomnia, and you have tried everything you can think of to remedy the difficulty without success, you may wish to put the above suggestion to the test. You certainly have nothing to lose and you may be delightfully surprised.

Postures for sleeping and relaxing

All yoga postures and breathing and meditation exercises have the potential for counteracting tension and fatigue, promoting rest and replenishing energy. Some, however, aim specifically at body-mind relaxation and sleep of the best quality. The Toe-to-top relaxation technique (Savasana) in chapter four is perhaps unsurpassed. It is usually practised in a supine position, that is, lying on the back, as illustrated in Fig. 33.

A variation of this posture, which may be practised in an easy chair, was described earlier in this chapter (the All-body Relaxation).

Another yoga relaxation posture, the Stick Posture, was described in chapter four as well. Instead of using it as an all-body stretch, you may simply rest in the position described: lie at full length on your back, with your arms extended above your head, and the palms of the hands turned upward. Separate your legs for maximum comfort. Breathe slowly and rhythmically.

At the slightest suggestion of strain on the lower back, modify the position, thus: bend your legs, place the soles of the feet flat on the surface on which you are lying, a comfortable distance from your bottom, and lean one knee against the other. Experiment until you find the position that's best for you.

The Crocodile Posture (also called the Dolphin Posture) is done lying face downward, stretched out at full length, somewhat like a prone version of the Stick Posture. You may adjust your head for ease of breathing, and your arms and legs for maximum comfort. Turn the palms of your hands downward. Remember to practise slow, rhythmic breathing.

Note

In chapter two, I mentioned that, generally, it is not a good idea to lie prone; certainly not for long periods. Some people, however, find the face downward positions relaxing when practised for short periods.

When lying prone, therefore, it's a good idea to place a thin cushion or folded towel under your hips, to prevent accentuation of the arch of the lower spine, and strain of the back muscles.

A variation of the Crocodile Posture is to position your arms alongside your body, rather than stretched out ahead. This then becomes somewhat of a prone equivalent of Savasana (Fig. 33). Do adjust your head position for comfort and ease of breathing.

Side Relaxation Posture

This posture is reminiscent of the lying position illustrated in Fig. 16, in chapter two. In this instance, however, there are modifications: if you lie on your left side, for instance, you fold your left arm and rest your head on your left palm. Your right leg rests on top of the left, both slightly bent for maximum comfort. The right arm rests at the right side of the body, either on the right thigh or placed beside the left arm.

Reverse the instructions if you lie on your right side. Also, remember to keep the spine well aligned and to breathe slowly and rhythmically.

The foregoing postures are suitable for brief periods of relaxation. For longer periods of rest and sleep, the lying positions described in chapter two (Figs. 15 and 16) may be more appropriate. Do experiment with the various positions to find those that are best for you.

Herbal remedies

Infusions of sedative herbs such as catmint, chamomile flowers, dill, hops, lime blossom, melitot, passion flower, sage and valerian will help calm you down and promote a pleasant drowsiness.

Make the infusion as you would brew ordinary tea, generally using one teaspoon of the herb to a cup of water. Drink a cupful of the beverage shortly before going to bed. You may sweeten the drink with a little unpasteurized honey, if you wish.

Another herbal tea you can try is this: add a pinch of lime flowers, a pinch of marjoram and a pinch of vervain to a cupful of hot water. Let the herbs infuse for a few minutes. Strain the tea and sip it slowly, sweetened or unsweetened.

Hops pillows

Hops pillows are an old standby for problem sleepers. To make a pillow, sew together two squares of fabric (the measurements depend on the size of pillow you wish; a small one is adequate).

Fill the pillow with hops cones. If you find the scent overpowering, add other herbs such as lavender or rose petals, with emphasis on the hops.

As you breathe in the scent of the hops, you will become drowsy and fall asleep.

Herbal baths

A warm bath containing an infusion of hops (and other herbs if you wish) taken shortly before slipping into a warm bed will promote recuperative sleep.

A bath containing essential oils, such as those from hops, orange blossom and meadowsweet, can also be wonderfully relaxing.

It is often the fear of insomnia rather than the sleeplessness itself that produces the deleterious effects of a poor night's rest. Don't let sleep obsess you to the point where, if you miss an hour or half an hour of it, you regard it as a calamity.

Follow the suggestions in this chapter, and anything else you consider useful to promote adequate sleep. If everything tried is to no avail, however, *seek a doctor's advice*. If he or she prescribes medication, take it but continue practising the relaxation techniques in this book.

Using your head to save your back

Stress has become a household word. It is something without which we cannot live. It is what enables some individuals to achieve great things. When stress is continuous and unrelieved, however, it becomes a destructive force. It produces unnecessary tension which can spread and cause discomfort, aches and pain. It can drain our energy and make us feel exhausted. Stress detracts from the joy of living.

What is stress?

Stress occurs when the demands of our internal or external environment, or both, tax or overwhelm our personal resources for dealing with them.

Effects of stress

Stress brings about undesirable changes in the structure and function of body tissues. These changes are largely responses to hormones secreted by glands located above the kidneys (the adrenal glands). They include:

● increased pulse rate;

● elevated blood pressure;

● faster rate of breathing;

● temporary impairment of digestion;

● withdrawal of mineral from bones;

● mobilization of fat from storage deposits;

● retention of an abnormal amount of salt in the body.

Stressors

A stressor is something that generates stress. It may be an event, a circumstance or some other agent. How it affects you depends essentially on how *you* perceive it. One person may regard a certain incident as comical and laugh about it. Another individual may look at the same occurrence and be offended or distressed by it, and for the latter individual that occurrence may be stressful.

Types of stressors

Stressors can take the form of everyday irritations in our relationship with others: spouse, children, acquaintances and co-workers. Some stressors are more short term yet more powerful ~ like a bereavement. All these stressors take a toll on our system, and all have the potential to produce chronic problems, to deplete our energy and to undermine our health.

Notorious stressors include apprehension, anxiety, fear, guilt, conflict, regret and uncertainty. These are all negative emotions that eventually compromise our health.

Another well-recognized stressor is having too many life changes occur in too short a period of time, for instance, losing one's job, moving house, starting a new career, and starting a new relationship, all in the same year. Experts predict that this increases the risk of a serious illness or accident, and I have seen their prediction come to pass again and again.

Control is the secret

Stressors lose their impact when they cease to deprive you of a sense of control. Once you learn to view an event, circumstance or other potential stressor as something over which you *do* have a measure of control, and which is not going to last forever, you have made an important first step in effective stress management.

Strategies for effective stress control

Information is the first step toward effective stress management. Be informed, so as to equip yourself to combat harmful stressors.

Keeping fit is an essential second step toward effective stress control. All the exercises ~ physical, breathing and medi-tative ~ in this book will contribute to your keeping fit. The nutrition information in chapter three will be useful as well to help you provide your body with the correct nutritive material for peak fitness.

The third positive step toward intelligent stress control is to establish and maintain a reliable emotional support system. This could be a trusted, dependable friend or group of friends or a professional counsellor with whom you have a good rapport. A good support system will provide you with encouragement when you feel discouraged and will furnish you with a safe, healthy outlet for feelings that need to be expressed rather than suppressed. A good support system will, moreover, reinforce positive feelings and promote a sense of self-worth and self-confidence, which are often almost destroyed when you feel despondent. Again and again, research has shown that stifling emotions results in hurt to oneself rather than to others.

To complement the three foregoing main stress management strategies, here are others suggested by various experts on stress:

- During the first few unpleasant moments of a stressful situation try this: smile inwardly and also with your eyes and mouth to reduce facial tension. Take a smooth, slow, deep breath in, and then exhale steadily while letting go of tightness from your jaws, tongue and shoulders. Mentally tell yourself that you are calm, alert and in control.

- Learn to identify and to anticipate both internal and external sources of stress.

- Learn to recognize symptoms of stress, such as a racing heartbeat or heart palpitations, irritability, anxiety, diarrhoea, tight jaws, and a tense back.

- Regularly practise a relaxation technique you enjoy and find effective. I have described some in detail earlier in this chapter, and also in chapter four. Regular practice of a relaxation technique will provide you with a break from routine activities and help you replenish your energy supplies. It will help reduce the impact of stressful stimuli and allow you time to recover. It will enable you to become more in touch with yourself and thus better able to recognize symptoms of stress.

- Have some fun. Psychologists and psychiatrists agree that play is very important for well-being. Balance work with a hobby or sport you enjoy. Avoid bringing to your recreation the spirit of competition or the compulsion to win. Play for pleasure.

- Delegate chores so that you are not overburdened. Learn to say 'no' without feeling guilty when this is appropriate. This prevents overcommitment. Learn how to be assertive yet gracious.

- Learn to laugh. Laughter is one of the best medicines you can take and it has no adverse effects.

- Practise not giving to the others the power to make you react before you are completely prepared to act (review the first of the above stress management suggestions).

Work strategies

Effective time management is an essential part of stress management. Aches and pain in the neck and back are sometimes a manifestation of continual hard mental and/or physical work without the balancing effects of adequate rest and relaxation, regular exercise and adequate nutrition. Backache and related symptoms are sometimes a consequence of working hard rather than working intelligently.

Here are some tips from experts on making the best of available time so you don't become overstressed, wondering how you're going to find time to do all you have and want to do:

- Keep fit. Back problems, lack of energy and illness result in poor work performance and absenteeism.

- Reduce clutter. When in doubt, throw it out! Reduce paper waste; use the telephone when you can. If you haven't used an item for years, consider giving it to a charitable organization or discard it.

- Shorten tea and coffee breaks. Use such breaks for rest from routine chores and for refreshment; not for prolonged socializing. Try taking a 'yoga break' and practising some of the local relaxation techniques described in chapter four. You can also practise breathing exercises during your breaks.

- Profit from travel time. If you have to travel to and from your place of work, find ways to use the time constructively. Listen to a cassette to help you improve skills related to your work or to further inform you about ways of coping with stress. Practise 'en route' exercises, such as described in chapter nine.

- Plan your work. Management efficiency experts emphasize that time spent planning is not wasted. Planning, in fact, saves time in the long term.

- Learn to concentrate. Inability to concentrate results in time wasted through having to backtrack and undo or re-do projects. Inability to concentrate can also lead to injury and accidents. Try practising, on a regular basis, the concentration techniques described earlier in this chapter.

- Control interruptions. Learn to protect your prime time. Unplug your telephone or let your answering machine take your calls. Catch up on work when others are on their breaks. It's not time itself that's significant to the successful completion of a project; it's the amount of *uninterrupted* time.

- Don't procrastinate. Explore why you tend to procrastinate; there may be underlying psychological reasons. Ask yourself why you're putting off that job. Ask what benefits you would derive if you were to tackle it promptly and finish it. The answer may help you overcome the delays.

- Avoid perfectionism. It's impossible to achieve perfection, in most cases, and it's frustrating to attempt to do so. Frustration is a stressor. Aim instead for excellence of effort and performance.

- Shorten telephone calls. Most phone calls, incoming and outgoing, can be shortened without disaster. Try this: time all calls for the next week or so. Record their length. Try ways of shortening them.

- Cut down on television viewing. Unless a programme entertains or enlightens you, consider not watching it. Read instead, or play word games (or other games) in which family members can participate. The time spent with family will enhance interpersonal relationships and contribute to the support system mentioned in the section on stress management.

- Don't be a workaholic. It takes intelligence and discernment to distinguish between activities that bring positive results and those that simply help pass the time away. The antidote for workaholism is not to work harder, but to be more organized.

- Don't be too houseproud. Keep the home reasonably clean and tidy. Practise 'minimal maintenance'. Rather than have an exhausing major cleanup once a month, for example, clean one room today, another tomorrow and another the next day. Enlist help from family members. Delegate chores.

- Relax! Backache and back pain and associated fatigue are prime timewasters. Incorporate simple relaxation techniques into your work day. The warm-ups in chapter four and the breathing exercises in this chapter are examples of suitable techniques you can weave into daily schedules.

Chapter 9

Back Talk for Special Needs

In the introduction to this book I remarked that almost everyone will experience some form of backache or pain or related symptom at some time. There are those of us, however, who are more susceptible to back problems because of the type of occupation in which we're regularly engaged, or sport in which we habitually participate.

It would be impossible to include all activities and conditions that put the back at risk. I have, however, selected some I consider particularly noteworthy, and these follow.

Back Talk for Sportspeople

Although the spine is not the most frequently injured part of the body in athletes, epidemiologic studies indicate that it sustains a high proportion of the most serious injuries (Nicholas and Hershman, 1172).

The spine provides the support and balance essential to stance and to the active motions of sports, such as running, jumping and kicking.

Sports most often associated with spinal injury include gymnastics, football, racquet sports, diving, horseback riding, trampolining and rugby. Racquet sports such as tennis and squash apply substantial torque

and rotational force to the spine. In golf, the twisting motion accompanying the drive is the risky part of the sport, since it can damage the intervertebral discs and the facet joints. These motions are often complex and involve sudden changes in direction.

As the spine ages, injuries tend to be of a more chronic and degenerative nature, and it becomes more important than before to pay special attention to any existing weakness, contracture or imbalance, as well as to one's endurance. Many older people who go skiing, for example, have some form of degenerative bone disorder, such as osteoporosis. If you are one of these individuals, you should take extreme care since breaks will occur far more easily than if you were younger.

Even young athletes are not exempt from back problems. Those with weak abdominals and tight hamstrings may be candidates for spinal injuries. Chapter six offers effective exercises for improving abdominal muscle tone, while chapter seven is devoted to exercises for the leg muscles.

There is no doubt whatever that those who are in peak physical condition are less liable to sustain injuries during sporting activities than those who are not.

Occasional athletes usually comprise the bulk of sports participants. These athletes spend most of the week in sedentary occupations, and play tennis or go horseback riding on weekends. For both men and women in this group, conditioning is particularly important. In addition, a period of training is essential to develop the muscles used in the particular sport engaged in, and to maintain that muscular development. You must have a warm-up period before participating in your chosen sport (see chapter four), and your body weight should be controlled (review chapter three).

If you are recovering from a spinal injury, it is very important to refrain from activities that subject the spine to torque and rotational force (such as racquet sports) until an orthopaedic physician has assessed the damage and given you permission to resume them. Rehabilitation exercise such as walking, cycling and swimming is often recommended during the convalescent period.

Low back pain in athletes

About three out of five athletes who experience low back pain state that their pain appears after they have participated in a sport or similar activity. Robin McKenzie, an internationally known consultant physiotherapist, has remarked that the true cause of pain in many of these individuals is the adoption of a slouched position following a thorough exercising of the joints involved.

During vigorous exercise, the joints of the spine are moved vigorously in many directions over an extended period of time. This causes thorough stretching in all directions of the soft tissues surrounding the joints. Moreover, the fluid gel content of the spinal discs (see chapter one) is loosened, and it would appear that distortion or displacement can occur if exercised joints are subsequently placed in an extreme posture, such as collapsing in a heap or slouching.

McKenzie's advice for athletes and others who engage in vigorous activity, and who have recently developed low back pain, is to try to expose the true cause of the problem.

It is necessary to determine whether the pain appears during a particular activity or afterwards. If the pain appears during the activity, then the sport itself may be the cause of the problem.

To ascertain if low back pain is the result of slouched sitting after participating in a sport or other vigorous activity, observe your posture carefully and sit correctly, with the low back in moderate lordosis (curving towards the front), supported by a lumbar roll if necessary (see chapter two). This means not sinking into a 'comfortable' chair or slouching in a car after, say, having played a few sets of tennis or a round of golf. It means sitting with meticulous attention to good posture (please review chapter two). Should pain occur following this careful attention to posture, then the cause is probably due to the sport in which you're involved, or the way you practise it. It would then be a good idea to have this looked into.

Lumbar Lessons Behind the Wheel

Studies indicate that the incidence of low back injuries is on the increase, and experts point out that spinal problems can be induced by stresses incurred through lack of awareness of the spine's limitations. They suggest that many of these can be prevented through a better understanding of the structure and function of the spine (see chapter one) and of good body mechanics (see chapter two).

There are other measures motorists can take to protect their back and avoid needless suffering, inconvenience and expense. Here are some examples.

● Adjust the seat of your vehicle so that your legs can reach the pedals without being locked straight. Relax your knee joints.

- Sit as far back in your seat as you comfortably can, keeping your spine well aligned, with your ears in line with your shoulders. Maintain an upright, but *not* rigid posture. Relax your shoulders and your jaws. Breathe regularly.

- If necessary, support your back with a special back support, which some motor supplies stores sell; or try to obtain a lumbar roll (*see* chapter two). This prop will help protect your spine from the ill effects of side-to-side jostling when you drive over bumps or make turns.

- Don't clutch the steering-wheel like a weapon. This promotes tension. Hold it securely but in a relaxed manner.

Whether you're behind the wheel or are engaged in other activities, the way you hold and carry yourself, as well as the way you perform various movements, will affect the health of your back, and indeed your overall health. Many people experience pains and muscle spasms because they do not sit, stand, lie or work with their bodies properly aligned. When for example, we slouch at the wheel, we cramp organs and blood vessels. Our lungs can't expand fully and so the intake of oxygen, which is vital to body cells (particularly those of the brain) is inadequate. We begin to feel low in energy; we can't think clearly, concentrate properly or react spontaneously. We subject spinal muscles to greater than normal strain and promote aches and pain. With pain comes depression, and a vicious circle is created.
Here are further tips on posture.

- Sit on the 'sitting bones' (one under each buttock), rather than on the end of your spine. When not driving, try to rest your feet on a prop so that your knees are higher than your hips. This relaxes the back muscles.

- When walking to and from your vehicle, or elsewhere develop the habit of walking tall to reduce stress. Tighten your abdomen and buttocks so as to reduce the arch in the lower back. (The parts of the intervertebral discs within the spinal curves receive more pressure than those on the outside of the curves. They are therefore subjected to more wear and tear.) If you practise keeping your pelvis tilted somewhat backward, it will reduce the lower back curve and help prevent disc problems. Please review good posture in standing, Figs. 13 and 14 in chapter two.

- Stand as little as possible. In many non-industrialized societies, people generally stand only to move from one place to another. When they wish to chat, they squat (*see* Fig. 10, chapter two). Squatting reduces accentuated spinal curves, thus relieving stress on intervertebral discs, and gives back muscles a therapeutic stretch. There is a notable absence of back problems among people who habitually squat.

- Lorry (truck) drivers often take time off for a nap in their vehicles during long journeys. Other long-distance motorists lie down for half an hour or so when they begin to tire. Apply the squatting principle when lying: lie on your side; bend your hips and knees. Bring your lower knee closer to your chest than your upper knee. Arrange your arms for comfort. (*See also* Fig. 16, chapter two).

- Avoid overweight. Excess weight places unnecessary strain on the spine and related structures. Review chapter three for information on nutrition.
A rigid spine is more vulnerable to strains and injuries than a flexible one. Following are suggestions for some pleasant, easy-to-do little exercises you can try in a variety of places, such as at rest stops along the way.

- *Warm-ups.* Always warm up before exercising to avoid pulls and strains. Stand tall. Put your hands on your hips or stretch them sideways or in front of you. Inhale and rise onto your toes (hold on to a stable prop if you need to). Exhale and lower yourself to a squatting position. Inhale and come up to a standing position, on your toes. Repeat the up-and-down movement several times in succession, synchronizing breathing with movement. Rest.

This warm-up is excellent for keeping the hip, knee and ankle joints flexible, to facilitate squatting.

Practise the ankle, neck and shoulder warm-ups in chapter four.

● Practise the Posture Clasp (Fig. 11) and the Chest Expander (Fig. 12) in chapter two.

● Practise the Pelvic Tilt, in any convenient position (see chapter five).

● Use your breath as a resource during stressful times on the road. Inhale slowly, smoothly and deeply through your nostrils. Exhale through pouted lips, as if cooling a hot beverage or whistling a tune. Repeat the exercise several times in smooth succession.

Even slowing down your breathing, and making it smooth and deep can have a calming effect when you feel tension mounting as you drive. Remember to let go of tightness in your lips and jaws and to relax your other facial muscles.

● Using a seat belt with both chest and lap components gives protection to both the dorsal and lumbar spine. A properly designed headrest will give protection to the cervical spine.

Menstruation

Backache can occur both premenstrually and during the menstrual period itself. It is important to know if your backache is cyclic, or if it may be attributed to some other condition. If you have any doubt whatever

that your backache is related to your menstrual cycle, you should have a general physical and pelvic examination by your doctor to exclude any medical or gynaecological condition, such as lupus (dealt with later in this chapter), fibroids or endometriosis.

Once it has been determined that your backache or back pain is a symptom of PMS (Premenstrual Syndrome) or dysmenorr-hoea (painful menstrual period), there are several things you can do to ease the discomfort. You can

● rest in bed in a position you find most comfortable (see chapter two for suggestions), with a heating pad or hot-water bottle, duly protected, applied to the affected part for short periods. (Sometimes local heat, used for prolonged periods, can increase pelvic congestion and therefore pain.)

● Try to practise a breathing or relaxation technique, such as those described in chapter eight. It is sometimes difficult to do this when you are in pain, but the effort is worthwhile. Tension and anxiety do increase pain (see chapter eight). You might try the modified version of Savasana and any of the breathing exercises described in chapter eight.

● Pay attention to your posture and carriage, as well as to your work habits. Good posture and body mechanics are important to backache prevention, as emphasized throughout this book. Please review chapter two.

● When not in pain, exercises to practise regularly for backache prevention include Squatting (Fig. 10, chapter two), the Lying Twist (Fig. 22), the Cobra (Fig. 30), both in chapter four, the Cat Stretch series (Figs. 34 to 37), the Pelvic Tilt (Figs. 38 and 39), the Bridge (Fig. 40), the Knee Presses (Figs. 41 to 43), the Star Posture (Fig. 44), the Pose of a Child (Fig. 45) and its variation described in chapter seven, following the Half-Locust, the Spinal Twist (Fig. 47), all to be found in chapter five, the Single Leg Raise (Fig. 51) and variations in chapter six, and the Half-Locust.

Remember to warm up properly before practising these and other exercises. Please review chapter four.

Here's another exercise you can add to your repertoire for helping prevent backache and back pain before and during your period.

The Spread-leg Stretch

1. Sit naturally erect on your mat, with your legs stretched out in front of you and spread apart as widely as is absolutely comfortable. Rest your palms on your legs. Breathe regularly.

2. Exhale and bend forward, at the hip joints rather than at the waist, sliding your hands down your legs.

3. When you can bend no farther, hold the position for several seconds. Do *not* hold your breath. Keep breathing regularly.

4. Inhale and slide your hands backward along your legs as you resume your starting position.

5. Place your hands on the mat beside you, bend your legs and assume a folded-legs position and rest; or lie down and relax.

One other measure to try for back relief is a sitz bath. If you don't have a special sitz tub, improvise. Fill a large, deep basin with enough warm water so that when you sit in it your pelvis is submerged. (The water temperature should be between 38° and 46°C, that is, between 100° and 115°F.) Add more warm water to maintain this temperature, if necessary.

Ideally, your feet should not be in the water, which makes a basin more suitable than a bathtub.

Remain in the sitz bath for ten to twenty minutes, and keep your upper body warm.

For more information on natural ways to overcome menstrual problems, read my book entitled *Pain-free Periods* (*see* bibliography).

Pre- and Post-natal Back Chat

The not uncommon occurrence of backache in pregnancy is due, in part, to an altered centre of gravity and consequent increased lordosis (forward spinal curvature in the lumbar region), as well as to a relaxing of joints due to hormonal influences. There's also fatigue, which deters effort at maintaining good habits. Strict attention to good posture (*see* chapter two) is, however, of the utmost importance, to prevent strains, aches and pain. Keeping good abdominal muscle tone (*see* chapter six) is crucial, as well, for keeping back problems to a minimum both pre- and post-natally. The back exercises in chapter five are useful, with modifications where necessary, to suit your own situation. Remember to warm up adequately (*see* chapter four) before exercising.

Here are additional tips for pregnant women and those who have recently given birth.

● *Don't* wear high heels. It encourages poor posture. It aggravates the arch in your lower back and increases strain on spinal supports. Wearing high heels leads to a shortening of the hamstring muscles which, as mentioned in chapter one, are secondary back supports contributing to the tilt of the pelvis. High heels, moreover, put too much weight on the front part of the foot, and if the toes of the shoes are narrow, they make foot muscles rigid and tense. This, in turn, leads to tense leg muscles which promote tension of the back muscles.

- Tight stockings or tights are also bad for the back. They interfere with the relaxation of the toes and feet which, as just mentioned, have a bearing on how the back feels.

- Brassieres with narrow straps can cause aches in the shoulders and upper back, partly because of direct pressure and partly because of the rigid position into which they force the wearer. Both contribute to back tension.

- Make sure your work surfaces in the kitchen are of the right height for *you*: They should be about 5 to 7 cm (2 to 3 inches) lower than your elbows to that you don't have to stoop. Stand as close as you can to the work area and, if possible, rest your hips against it.

- When you must stand, try resting one foot on a low stool, a foot-rail or other prop about 10 to 15 cm (4 to 6 inches) above the floor. This will relax the psoas muscle, which stretches from the lower back across the pelvis to the thigh, and relieve strain on the back.

Caesarean Section

Most women who have had a caesarean delivery are up and about the day after surgery. Early, graduated, consistent exercise is very important to the healing process and to promote proper union of the incision edges. It is also essential to help restore muscle tone and function of all body structures.

Since the abdominal muscles give reinforcement to the back (*see* chapter six), it is important that these be quickly strengthened through appropriate exercise. Start with a simple breathing technique. While lying comfortably, support your abdomen with your hands. Take a slow, smooth, deep breath in through your

nostrils. Exhale steadily through your mouth while saying 'huh' or 'huff'.

Repeat this exercise several times in succession. Don't be afraid that your stitches will pop; they won't.

Progress to simple leg exercises. From a supine position, with the small of your back firmly pressed to the surface on which you are lying, and with legs straight ahead, slide one heel toward you then away from you, several times in slow succession. Repeat the exercise with the other leg. Remember to keep breathing regularly.

As your strength and energy return, work slowly up to the exercises in chapters five, six and seven. Always warm up first (*see* chapter four). Also recommended is the practice of breathing exercises and some form of meditation every day. Suggestions are given in chapter eight.

For more in-depth information on keeping fit during and after pregnancy, you may wish to look at my book entitled *Easy Pregnancy with Yoga* (see bibliography).

Beating Back Fatigue

There are several conditions that cause sufferers to feel low in energy generally, and to experience back fatigue not infrequently. The first that comes to mind is M.E. (myalgic encephalomyelitis), also referred to as C.F.S. (chronic fatigue syndrome). This is a condition in which normal body and central nervous system functions have been disturbed and deranged. There are two schools of thought as to the causes: one is that of persistent viral infection due to non-effectiveness of normal immune mechanism; the other is that persisting viral infection triggers an abnormal immune response. Whatever the cause or causes of M.E. are, fatigue is one of the most frequent symptoms.

S.L.E. (systemic lupus erythematosus, or 'lupus') is another disorder that tends to curtail activity. Lupus is sometimes classified as an auto-immune disease, in which the body turns on itself, as it were. It is also described as a collagen disease. Collagen is the cement-like material that holds body cells together (*see* chapter one). Anything affecting the integrity of the body's collagen will cause it to weaken. People with lupus often report persisting aches and pains in joints of the back and elsewhere, and they tend to tire easily.

Yet another debilitating condition is M.S. (multiple sclerosis), a chronic progressive nervous system disease of unknown cause. Many people with M.S. function seemingly normally, but as the disease advances, energy is affected and mobility restricted.

As we age, too, we tend to feel fatigue more readily than when we were younger. Also, we may not be as mobile or active. Often, the back is the first place where we feel the symptoms of ageing.

Fatigue is a warning symptom. It signals that the body is tired and should be rested. To ignore this warning is to court trouble in the form of pain or injury. When your back is tired, you need to rest it. It's that simple. You will find the lying positions described in chapter two (Figs. 15 and 16), the Pose of a Child (Fig. 45, chapter five) and its variation in chapter seven are useful. You could also sit in a recliner (easy chair) that provides good support for your spine, arms and legs. While resting, practise a breathing or relaxation exercise such as described in chapters four and eight.

To strengthen the back, and the abdomen which gives reinforcement to the back muscles, practise the basic versions of the exercises in chapters five and six, making sure that you warm up properly, as suggested in chapter four. Keep your legs well toned by practising the exercises in chapter seven. Shortened hamstring muscles increase the arch of the lower back, thus imposing strain on back structures.

If you find some of the exercises too challenging for you, then omit them, or modify them to suit your particular state. The neck, shoulder and ankle warm-ups in chapter four are easy to do and help prevent tension from building up. The Pelvic Tilt and the Knee Presses in chapter five are not difficult. The Single Raise (chapter six) and the Butterfly (chapter seven) are also among the easier exercises you might wish to try.

Sex Without Back Pain

There are few illnesses that should be allowed to interfere totally with physical intimacy between two loving partners. Even if you don't feel well enough to engage in sexual intercourse, simply holding each other close can be a wonderful experience.

Various illnesses, such as those mentioned in the previous section, cause the sufferers to tire easily. They may produce stiffness and aching joints. They may cause pain. Even the fear of pain will decrease interest in sex: fear generates tension and tension can eventually produce pain.

People being treated with the drug cortisone tend to bruise easily and some develop painful hips. Cortisone also produces sexual apathy in some individuals. The bruising or fear of bruising may inhibit the desire for sex or make the other partner feel guilty about causing injury. One partner may sense the other's need for gratification but, feeling exhausted, is unable to meet this need. The other partner may feel denied or rejected.

In any case where there are factors that have the potential to damage sexual relationships, it is vitally important that the partners at least attempt to understand each other's feelings. It is essential that apprehensions, fears, feelings of guilt, etc., be sensitively discussed. Don't hesitate to seek professional help, if necessary. Reduced sexual ardour need not mean lack of love or interest, but this should be made clear.

Keep communication lines open. Make adjustments. Show consideration. Remember: having a chronic illness or growing older does not necessarily mean that sexual activity must be curtailed or eliminated.

Postural adjustments

Couples who have a warm, loving relationship will find ways over or around sexual obstacles. Orgasm, in fact, is said to trigger a release of natural cortisone, which can be helpful in reducing pain. (Cortisone is a hormone produced by the cortex, or outer portion, of the adrenal glands which are located above the kidneys.)

If your problem is facet joint strain, you are probably better off lying on your back, with your partner on top. If pain strikes during intercourse, try gentle pelvic tilting (*see* Fig. 39) to reduce the curve in your lower back and diminish strain on the joints.

The pelvic thrusting movements of sexual intercourse may work as a mobilizing exercise when you lie supine. These are reminiscent of the Pelvic Tilt (Fig. 39). Your knees should be bent and your feet placed flat on the bed or wherever you are lying. If you assume an all-fours position, with your partner behind you, the pelvic rocking movements are similar to the Cat Stretch (Fig. 34). Be careful not to accentuate the concave arch of the back. The all-fours position is also worth a try if you like lying on your back but your partner is much heavier than you.

Another position for women to try is one reminiscent of the Knee Press, Variation II (*see* chapter 5, Fig. 43), omitting step 4 of the instructions, and keeping the head flat. The partner kneels, and the woman is thus spared the weight of the man's body. She can support her bent legs or her partner can. A little experimentation and creativity will quickly teach both partners the best arrangement for them.

If you both have back problems, try lying side by side, arranging your limbs for maximum comfort.

A man with back pain may be more comfortable sitting in a chair than lying down. The female partner can then sit astride him and be the more active participant. Here, too, the pelvic tilting exercise comes in handy.

The following is a little exercise which, although not involving the back muscles, is useful for women to practise regularly. It tones up the perineum, which is the lowest part of the torso, between the legs, thus improving support for pelvic organs.

Breathe regularly. On an *exhalation*, tighten your vagina and anus. Hold the tightness until your exhalation is complete. Inhale and relax. Repeat the exercise once now and again later.

You can do this perineal exercise almost anywhere because no one can see what you are doing. You can do it during sex to enhance your partner's pleasure.

Other exercises to practise regularly to keep you fit for sex include the Lying Twist (Fig. 22), the Cat Stretch series (Figs. 35 to 37), the Bridge (Fig. 40), the Butterfly (Fig. 53) and the Spread-leg Stretch described in this chapter in the section entitled 'Menstruation'.

Modify any or all of these exercises to suit your particular situation.

Check local libraries and bookstores for books about fostering mutually satisfying sexual relationships. Some are specially written for people with mobility difficulties. All emphasize the importance of good communication through talking, listening, touching and other forms of tenderness. Also check community services for leaflets on this subject.

Backup

Doctors and other health professionals emphasize personal responsibility in caring for your back. They stress the importance of putting good postural habits into daily practice, and of exercising faithfully in order to control back problems so that those problems don't control *you*.

The background information presented in this book, along with exercise instructions and illustrations will provide you with basic resources for looking after your back with intelligence. The additional hints to follow will supplement the information given in preceding chapters.

● If you feel a back spasm coming, lie on the floor, with a cushion under your head and buttocks for support, and rest your legs on a chair. Position your buttocks as far under the chair as possible so that your trunk is at right angles to your thighs.

● If you hurt your back, apply an ice pack to the sore area for about fifteen minutes every four to six hours. This will anaesthetize the affected part, minimize inflammation and pain and prevent further swelling.

● If your back becomes stiff, try heat. A heating pad or hot-water bottle (properly covered) applied to the stiff area, or taking a hot bath or shower will bring some relief.

● Massage is often wonderful for a sore back. It helps increase blood flow to the hurting area, relax the muscles and decrease pain.

● When muscles or joints are inflamed and painful, they must be adequately rested to ease discomfort and permit healing.

● Avoid crossing your legs. It tilts the pelvis too far forward and increases lordosis.

This puts strain on the back. Whenever you sit on a chair, try to have your knees level with or slightly higher than your hips.

● If you must read in bed, sit upright and place a pillow under your knees to counteract strain on the lower back. If you read lying down, the strain on your neck can lead to degenerative changes in the cervical spine, and to arthritis and pain.

● Carry a baby as close as possible to your body or against your shoulder.

● Don't bend over to make a bed. Rest one bent knee on the bed, if you can, and brace yourself with your hand to ease pressure on your back.

● Support your abdomen with your hands when you cough or sneeze.

● Don't overload your briefcase.

● Keep luggage to a minimum and make it lightweight. Buy luggage with shoulder-straps.

● Find ways to exercise during the course of your day's work: deliver memos from office to office whenever you can; walk up and down stairs instead of using the lift (elevator); park your car well away from your destination so that you have to walk. The exercise will burn up excess adipose tissue, improve blood circulation and muscle tone and maintain good mobility. All these are essential to a healthy spine.

● Squat to put away papers in filing cabinets or to retrieve them; don't bend over.

● Remember the five back basics: regular exercise; proper body mechanics; adequate rest; good nutrition and weight control, and effective stress management.

Glossary

Anaesthetize
Make insensible to pain.

Articulation
The place of union between two or more bones; a joint.

Cervical
Pertaining to the region of the neck.

Collagen
A fibrous insoluble protein found in connective tissue, including bone, ligaments and cartilage.

Cyclic
Periodic; occurring in cycles.

Disc
See Intervertebral disc.

Dorsal
Pertaining to the back.

End plate
A layer of cartilage covering the upper and lower surfaces of intervertebral discs.

Facets
Bony surfaces on the rear part of a vertebra which match up with similar surfaces on the neighbouring vertebrae and guide their movements.

Facet joints
Joints formed by vertebral facets (*see* above).

Gynaecologic
Pertaining to the study of diseases peculiar to women.

Hamstrings
Three muscles on the back of the thigh. They flex the leg and adduct (bring toward the midline) and extend the thigh.

Immune
Protected against disease.

Immune response
The reaction of the body to substances that are foreign or interpreted as foreign.

Intervertebral disc
Broad, flattened disc of fibrocartilage between the bodies of vertebrae.

Kyphosis
Refers to a spinal curve that is convex toward the rear.

Lordosis
Refers to a spinal curve that is convex toward the front. The normal curve of the lumbar region of the spine is lordotic.

Lymph
An alkaline fluid found in lymphatic vessels.

Matrix (bone)
The intercellular substance from which bone develops.

Prone
Lying horizontal with the face downward. Opposite of supine.

Quadriceps
A large muscle on the front of the thigh.

Respiration
The act of breathing; inhaling and exhaling.

Sacral
Pertaining to the sacrum, a triangular bone located at the back of the pelvis. It is made up of five fused vertebrae.

Sacroiliac joints
The joints formed by the hip bones and the sacrum.

Skeletal
Pertaining to the body's bony framework.

Supine
Lying on the back, with the face upward. Opposite of prone.

Thoracic
Pertaining to the chest.

Torque
A force producing rotary motion.

Vertebra (pl. vertebrae)
Any one of the 33 bones forming the spinal column.

Vertebral column
Spine or spinal column. Backbone.

Viscera
Organs enclosed within a cavity, especially the abdominal organs.

Bibliography

Abraham, Edward A., MD, *Freedom from Back Pain. An Orthopedist's Self-Help Guide*, Emmaus, Pennsylvania: Rodale Press, 1986.

Airola, Paavo, Ph.D., *Dr Airola's Handbook of Natural Healing. How to Get Well*, Phoenix, Arizona: Health Plus Publishers, 1974.

Aladjem, Henrietta, *Understanding Lupus: What it is. How to treat it. How to cope with it*, New York: Charles Scribner's Sons, 1982.

Atkinson, Holly, MD, *Women and Fatigue*, New York: G.P. Putnam's Sons, 1985.

Benson, Herbert, *The Relaxation Response*, New York: William Morrow, 1975.

Brena, Steven F., MD, *Yoga and Medicine*, Baltimore, Maryland: Penguin Books, 1973.

Cailliet, Rene, MD, *Low Back Pain Syndrome* (3rd ed.), Philadelphia: F.A. Davis Company, 1981.

Caruth, Fran, and Thompson, Flora, *Transfer and Lifting Techniques for Extended Care*, Vancouver, Canada: 'Transfer Manual', P.O. Box 1341, Postal Station A, 1983.

Corbin, Dr Charles B., and Lindsey, Dr Ruth, *Concepts of Physical Fitness with Laboratories* (7th ed.), Dubuque, Iowa: Wm. C. Brown Publishers, 1991.

Davis, Adelle, *Let's Eat Right to Keep Fit*, New York: New American Library, 1970.

Deyo, Richard A., MD, MPH, 'Fads in the Treatment of Low Back Pain', *The New England Journal of Medicine*, Vol. 325, No. 14, Oct. 3, 1991, pp. 1039–1040.

Faelten, Sharon, and the Editors of Prevention Magazine, *The Complete Book of Minerals for Health*, Emmaus, Pennsylvania: Rodale Press, 1981.

Fahrni, W. Harry, MD, FRCS (Edinburgh), M.Ch. Orth. (Liverpool), *Backache Relieved Through New Concepts of Posture*, Springfield, Ill.: Charles C. Thomas, 1966.

Fine, Judylaine, *Conquering Back Pain. A Comprehensive Guide*, New York: Prentice Hall Press, 1987.

Fromm, Erich, *The Art of Loving*, New York: Bantam Books, 1963.

Gulledge, A. Dale, MD (Guest Ed.), 'Depression and Chronic Fatigue', *Primary Care. Clinics in Office Practice*, Vol. 18, No. 2, June 1991, Philadelphia: W.B. Saunders, 1991.

Hall, Hamilton, MD, *The Back Doctor*, Toronto: McClelland and Stewart-Bantam, 1980.

Hewitt, James, *The Complete Yoga Book*, New York: Schocken Books, 1977.

Hittleman, Richard, *Yoga: The 8 Steps to Health and Peace*, New York: Bantam Books, 1976.

Imrie, Dr David, and Barbuto, Dr Lu, *The Back Power Program*, Toronto: Stoddart Publishing, 1988.

Kaufmann, Klaus, *Silica. The Forgotten Nutrient*, Burnaby, Canada: Alive Books, 1990.

Kounovsky, Nicholas, *The Joy of Feeling Fit*, London: Pelham Books, 1971.

Kraus, Hans, MD, *Backache, Stress and Tension*, New York: Simon and Schuster, 1965.

Lagerwerff, Ellen B., and Perlroth, Karen A., *Mensendieck Your Posture and Your Pains*, New York: Anchor Press/Doubleday, 1973.

Lauersen, Niels H., MD, and Stukane, Eileen, *PMS. Premenstrual Syndrome and You*, New York: Pinnacle Books, 1983.

Leboyer, Frederick, *Birth Without Violence*, New York: Alfred A. Knopf, 1976.

Liang, Matthew H., MD (Guest Ed.), 'Musculoskeletal Pain Syndromes', *Primary Care. Clinics in Office Practice*, Vol. 15, No. 4, Dec. 1988. Philadelphia: W.B. Saunders, 1988.

Livingston, Michael, MD, *Beyond Backache. A Personal Guide to Back and Neck Pain Relief*, San Diego, California: Libra Publishers, 1988.

McKenzie, Robin, FNZSP, DIP, MT, *Treat Your Own Back* (4th ed.), Waikanae, New Zealand: Spinal Publications Ltd, 1988.

Mindell, Earl, *Earl Mindell's Pill Bible*, New York: Bantam Books, 1984.

Natow, Annette, and Heslin, Jo-Ann, *Nutrition for the Prime of Your Life*, New York: McGraw-Hill, 1983.

Nicholas, James A., and Hershman, Elliott B. (Eds), *The Lower Extremity and Spine in Sports Medicine*, Vol. 2, St. Louis: C.V. Mosby, 1986.

Noble, Elizabeth, RPT, *Essential Exercises for the Childbearing Year*, Boston: Houghton Mifflin, 1976.

Pelletier, Kenneth R., *Mind As Healer, Mind As Slayer*, New York: Dell Publishing, 1977.

Phillips, Robert H., Ph.D., *Coping With Lupus*, Wayne, New Jersey: Avery Publishing, 1984.

Schneider, Dr Johannes, 'Silica. A vital element for good health', *Alive Canadian Journal of Health & Nutrition*, No. 80, pp. 13–15.

Shreeve, Caroline M., MD, *The Alternative Dictionary of Symptoms and Cures*, London: Century Hutchinson, 1986.

Stanton, Rosemary, *Eating for Peak Performance*, Sydney: Allen & Unwin, 1988.

Stroebel, Charles F., MD, *QR The Quieting Reflex*, New York: Berkley Books, 1983.

Tanner, John, MB, BS, BSc., *Beating Back Pain. A Practical Self-Help Guide to Prevention and Treatment*, Toronto: Macmillan of Canada, 1988.

Tessman, Jack R., *My Back Doesn't Hurt Anymore*, New York: Quick Fox, 1980.

Turner, Roger Newman, B.Ac., N.D., D.O., M.R.O., *Banish Back Pain. Effective self-help with the aid of simple home remedies*, Wellingborough, England: Thorsons Publishers, 1989.

Van Straten, N.D., D.O., *The Complete Natural-Health Consultant*, New York: Prentice Hall Press, 1987.

Weller, Stella, *Easy Pregnancy with Yoga*, Wellingborough, England: Thorsons Publishing Group, 1991.

——, *Pain-free Periods*, Wellingborough, England: Thorsons Publishers, 1986.

——, 'Back Talk for Motorists', *Canadian Motorist*, November 1980, pp. 4-5, 12.

White, Augustus A. III, MD, *Your Aching Back. A Doctor's Guide to Relief*, New York: Bantam Books, 1983.

Workers' Compensation Board of British Columbia, *Back Talk. An Owner's Manual for Backs*, British Columbia, Canada: Workers' Compensation Board of Canada, 1987.

Yogendra, Sitadevi, Smt, *Yoga Simplified for Women*, Santa Cruz, Bombay: The Yoga Institute, 1972.

Index

By the same author . . .

Easy Pregnancy with Yoga

A welcome revised edition of this highly practical book, which contains essential information for helping the mother-to-be to enjoy a healthy pregnancy and to deliver her child confidently and naturally.

Yoga is a safe and relaxing exercise for pregnant women and the non-violent exercises (asanas) outlined in the book are practised in harmony with breathing techniques. Separate chapters cover body mechanics, deal with discomforts during pregnancy, preparing the breasts for breast feeding, and optimum nutrition during pregnancy. There are additional chapters on preparing for a caesarean birth and on restoring muscle tone and function quickly after the birth.

Illustrated with sixty drawings which complement the clear instructions, *Easy Pregnancy With Yoga* is an invaluable guide not only for mothers-to-be but also for health care professionals.

Of further interest . . .

Backache and Disc Troubles

The New Self Help series
Arthur White ND, DO

A vital self-help volume not only for those unfortunate enough to suffer already from back pain, but also for everyone aware of how important it is to protect what is literally the backbone of good health.

Arthur White, a naturopath:

- Pinpoints likely problem areas

- Explains the causes of back pain
- Offers effective strategies for alleviation and prevention of pain
- Provides guidance on lifestyle and nutrition
- Outlines a 'cleansing regime' and programme of remedial exercises

Thorsons Introductory Guide to Chiropractic

Dr Michael B. Howitt Wilson

Chiropractic is an increasingly popular specialist manipulative therapy, not unlike osteopathy, which pays special attention to the spine since the cause of many pain problems can be found there due to its very close relationship with the nervous system. It has been found to be particularly effective in dealing with back pain.

Dr Michael Howitt Wilson, a medical practitioner specializing in chiropractic treatment, gives an insight into the therapy, explains how it works and how it can help you.

A Gentler Strength

The yoga book for women

Paddy O'Brien

Yoga is an ideal exercise for women, helping rebalance stresses, explore conflicts about self-image and self esteem in a gentle untraumatic way. Yoga enhances flexibility, strength and power and gives women access to inner peace and tranquility.

A *Gentler Strength* is a book for women about the particular advantages and resources yoga has for them as a system of exercise and as an opportunity for development and exploration.

A *Gentler Strength* includes:

- A system of exercises that celebrate womanhood
- a basic yoga 'vocabulary' of postures and breathing
- a programme of postures for life passages from adolescence through pregnancy to old age
- illustrated with specially commissioned photographs and line drawings

Office Yoga

Tackling tension with simple stretches you can do at your desk

Julie Friedeberger

Office Yoga is a survival handbook for the desk-bound; a practical manual of simple movements which you can do a few minutes at a time throughout the day, to relieve the tension and stress of sedentary working life. It gives clear instructions and illustrations for sixty stretching and breathing exercises – simple, safe, and fun to do – most of which can be done sitting in your chair at your deak.

Doing Office Yoga will make you feel better. It will relieve and help prevent headache, neck-ache, back-ache and eye-ache. It will improve your vitality, boost your energy levels and improve your concentration.

Office Yoga also offers guidance on improving your personal working environment; chair, desk and lighting; and suggests how to make use of the time you spend travelling to and from work.

If you work at a desk, computer terminal or drawing board, in an office or at home, *Office Yoga* will be of sound, practical help to you.

EASY PREGNANCY WITH YOGA	0 7225 1931 1	£6.99	☐
NEW SELF-HELP BACKACHE & DISC TROUBLES	0 7225 1935 4	£2.99	☐
THORSONS INTRODUCTORY GUIDE TO CHIROPRACTIC	0 7225 2526 5	£3.99	☐
A GENTLER STRENGTH	0 7225 2536 2	£6.99	☐
OFFICE YOGA	0 7225 2537 0	£5.99	☐

All these books are available from your local bookseller or can be ordered direct from the publishers.

To order direct just tick the titles you want and fill in the form below:

Name: _____

Address: _____

_____

_____ Postcode: _____

Send to: Thorsons Mail Order, Dept 3, HarperCollins*Publishers*, Westerhill Road, Bishopbriggs, Glasgow G64 2QT.
Please enclose a cheque or postal order or your authority to debit your Visa/Access account —

Credit card no: _____

Expiry date: _____

Signature: _____

— up to the value of the cover price plus:
UK & BFPO: Add £1.00 for the first book and 25p for each additional book ordered.
Overseas orders including Eire: Please add £2.95 service charge. Books will be sent by surface mail but quotes for airmail despatches will be given on request.

24 HOUR TELEPHONE ORDERING SERVICE FOR ACCESS/VISA CARDHOLDERS — TEL: **041 772 2281.**